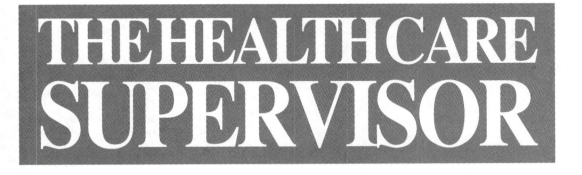

PRODUCTIVITY

Edited by
Charles R. McConnell
Vice President for Employee Affairs
The Genesee Hospital
Rochester, New York

AN ASPEN PUBLICATION®
Aspen Publishers, Inc.
Gaithersburg, Maryland
1993

Library of Congress Cataloging-in-Publication Data

The health care supervisor on productivity /
[edited by] Charles R. McConnell.
p. cm.
Includes bibliographical references and index.
ISBN: 0-8342-0368-5
1. Health facilities—Labor productivity. 2. Organizational effectiveness. I. McConnell, Charles R.
[DNLM: 1. Efficiency. 2. Health Services—organization & administration—United States. 3. Personnel Management. 4.
Health Facility Administrators.
WX 159 H4349 1993]
RA971.35.H427   1993
362.1'1'0685—dc20
DNLM/DLC
for Library of Congress
93-9324
CIP

Aspen Publishers, Inc. grants permission for photocopying for limited personal or internal use. This consent does not extend
to other kinds of copying, such as copying for general distribution, for advertising or promotional purposes, for creating new
collective works, or for resale. For information, address
Aspen Publishers, Inc., Permissions Department, 200 Orchard Ridge Drive, Suite 200,
Gaithersburg, Maryland 20878.

Editorial Resources: Barbara Priest

Library of Congress Catalog Card Number: 93-9324
ISBN: 0-8342-0368-5

Printed in Canada

1 2 3 4 5

Contents

Part I   Establishing Baselines

Part II   Tackling Productivity Improvement

Part III Involvement for Improvement

Part IV Other Dimensions of Productivity Improvement

Preface

INTRODUCTION

The Health Care Supervisor is a cross-disciplinary journal that publishes articles of relevance to persons who manage the work of others in health care settings. This journal's readers, as well as its authors, come from a wide variety of functional, clinical, technical, and professional backgrounds. Between the covers of a single issue of *HCS*, for example, you can find articles written by a nurse, a physician, a speech pathologist, a human resource specialist, an accountant, a nursing home administrator, and an attorney. These authors, and the numerous others who write for *HCS*, write with a single purpose: To provide guidance that all health care supervisors, regardless of the occupations or specialties they supervise, can use in learning to better understand or fulfill the supervisory role.

Productivity, in its simplest form is expressed as a relationship between the input to and output from some kind of system or activity. It is an ever-present concern of the supervisor. Unfortunately, however, the concept of productivity improvement cycles in and out of popularity with almost predictable frequency. Whether under the broad blanket of Total Quality Management or the narrower concept of Quality Circles, every now and then productivity improvement comes back around with all the trappings of a popular fad. And like a fad, it has its day and it is gone again without a great deal having changed.

Regardless of the prevailing notions concerning productivity, the supervisors who are most successful in the long run are the supervisors who by habit approach the work with a questioning attitude: Why do it this way?; Why not another way?; Why perform this step at all?; and so on, taking nothing for granted but constantly believing in the reality of continuing improvement.

In *The Health Care Supervisor on Productivity* we have assembled 19 articles that treat productivity with viewpoints ranging from the somewhat theoretical to the highly practical. Regardless of each author's individual direction, however, one common theme is clear: Productivity improvement is a constant responsibility and concern of the supervisor.

ESTABLISHING BASELINES

In establishing baselines for productivity improvement one decides what is to be improved, by how much, and why, and also determines what to measure change against. First, however, one buys into a belief in the value of productivity improvement. In "The Imperative of Assessment" Addison Bennett writes of the necessity to always examine how we do things in the belief that there can always be a better way. "Is Productivity Coming Into Its Own–Again?" suggests that the supervisor needs to look beyond the fad, past the gimmick, to see the true value of a belief in continuing improvement.

Scott MacStravic, in "Performance Auditing for Health Care Supervisors," suggests how to begin identifying our true improvement baseline by critically examining our own departmental activities. With "Work Smarter, Not Harder" Addison Bennett repeats some age-old but still valid advice concerning the need to think our problems through before acting.

The two final entries in this section, "Cost Containment: A New Way of Life" and "Survival Through Productivity Improvement" (Donald Beck and Jack Dempsey), raise the level of need for productivity improvement to one of urgency because of the increasingly restrictive environment in which today's health organizations must operate.

TACKLING PRODUCTIVITY IMPROVEMENT

In "Human Work Performance: It's Not as Simple As You Think" Richard Melecki suggests how to approach the broad issue of productivity by initially addressing the human element. Karen Zander, in "Revising the Production Process: When 'More' is Not the Solution," points out that the seemingly simple solution, to wring more output from the same input, is not often the preferred approach.

Three articles by John L. Templin, Jr., provide a primer of practical information about productivity for the supervisor. "Productivity and the Supervisor" defines productivity in its simplest terms and introduces the reader to productivity standards and their source, while "Productivity Monitoring for Every Supervisor" explains how to most easily track productivity in the department. "The Impact of Nonwidget-Producing Activities" highlights the need for attention to productivity in often overlooked service and support functions.

With "Work Simplification: A Supervisor's Challenge," Kenneth Cohen provides some solid advice as to how to begin changing the way things are done, for the purpose of instituting improvement.

INVOLVEMENT FOR IMPROVEMENT

In "Human Resource Management: Keystone for Productivity," Bruce Bartels and Keith Gee open up consideration of the critical need for employee involvement in productivity improvement. Dimensions of employee involvement are further explored by Robert Boissoneau in "The Importance of Japanese Management to Health Care Supervisors: Quality and American Circles," in "Quality Circles: A Supervisor's Tool for Solving Operational Problems in Nursing" by F. Theodore Helmer and Sarath Gunatilake, and by William Werther in "Involving Employees in Change, Productivity, and the Future." The common theme of these articles is founded in the sincere belief that complete success at productivity improvement depends on the direct involvement and participation of the employees who perform the work day-in and day-out.

OTHER DIMENSIONS OF PRODUCTIVITY IMPROVEMENT

Jerad Browdy advances the usefulness of incentive compensation in inspiring improved performance in "Incentive Compensation and the Health Care Super-visor." "Video Display Terminals: A New Source of Employee Problems" suggests that new technologies employed in productivity improvement bring with them new employee problems to be addressed. Finally, in "Improving Productivity in the Health Care Industry: An Argument and Supporting Evidence From One Hospital," Michael Koshuta and Michael McCuddy present some significant actual experience to demonstrate that productivity improvement can be a practical reality.

CONCLUSION

Thomas A. Edison was supposed to have said, "There's a way to do it better; find it." This admonition is strictly positive in tone, an imperative. It was not suggested that there *might* be, or there is *possibly*, or that *perhaps* there is a better way, or that we have any true alternatives to looking. In truth, Edison's statement sounds more like a command.

Indeed, virtually everything that humans do can be done better. If we fail to improve upon existing conditions it may mean that we are not yet intellectually or technologically equipped to go beyond the present; however, it most likely means that we have not really tried because we have not yet cared enough to look beyond the present.

In its finest form, productivity improvement springs from the kind of attitude reflected in Edison's statement. If we always believe there is a better way, we will eventually find it.

Acknowledgments

It would not have been possible to assemble this volume without the active involvement of the members of the guiding boards, past and present, of *The Health Care Supervisor*. As of this writing some of these valued advisors and authors are well into their second decade of service to *HCS*.

Our sincere thanks to the following past members of the *HCS* Editorial Board, the present *HCS* Advisory Board, and the present Board of Contributing Editors.

Past Members of *HCS* Editorial Board

Steven H. Appelbaum, Zeila W. Bailey, Claire D. Benjamin, Marjorie Beyers, Philip Bornstein, Leonard C. Brideau, Robert W. Broyles, Joy D. Calkin, Kenneth P. Cohen, Joseph A. Cornell, Darlene A. Dougherty, Kenneth R. Emery, Valerie Glesnes-Anderson, Lee Hand, Allen G. Herkimer, Jr., Max G. Holland, Bowen Hosford, Charles E. Housley, Loucine M. D. Huckabay, Laura L. Kalick, Janice M. Kurth, Marlene Lamnin, Joan Gratto Liebler, Ellyn Luros, Margeurite R. Mancini, Robert D. Miller, Joan F. Moore, Victor J. Morano, Harry E. Munn, Jr., Michael W. Noel, Rita E. Numerof, Samuel E. Oberman, Cheryl S. O'Hara, Jesus J. Pena, Donald J. Petersen, Tim Porter-O'Grady, George D. Pozgar, Ann Marie Rhodes, Edward P. Richards III, James C. Rose, Rachel Rotkovich, Norton M. Rubenstein, Edward D. Sanderson, William L. Scheyer, Homer H. Schmitz, Joyce L. Schweiger, Donna Richards Sheridan, Margaret D. Sovie, Eugene I. Stearns, Judy Ford Stokes, Thomas J. Tenerovicz, Lewis H. Titterton, Jr., Dennis A. Tribble, Terry Trudeau, Alex J. Vallas, Katherine W. Vestal, Judith Weilerstein, William B. Werther, Jr., Shirley Ann Wertz, Sara J. White, Norman H. Witt, and Karen Zander

Present *HCS* Advisory Board

Addison C. Bennett, Bernard L. Brown, Jr., Karen H. Henry, Norman Metzger, I. Donald Snook, Jr., and Helen Yura-Petro

Present Board of Contributing Editors

Donald F. Beck, Robert Boissoneau, Jerad D. Browdy, Vicki S. Crane, Carol A. Distasio, Charlotte Eliopoulos, Howard L. Lewis, R. Scott MacStravic, Leon McKenzie, Jerry L. Norville, Stephen L. Priest, Howard L. Smith, and John L. Templin, Jr.

Our sincere appreciation as well to those who, in addition to several persons mentioned above, participated in creating the articles that make up this present volume:

Bruce M. Bartels, Jack Dempsey, Keith L. Gee, Sarath Gunatilake, F. Theodore Helmer, Michael Koshuta, Michael K. McCuddy, and Richard G. Melecki.

Part I
Establishing Baselines

The imperative of assessment

Addison C. Bennett
Management Consultant
Los Angeles, California

ASSESSMENT—the act of evaluating the essential dimensions of current conditions and circumstances—is, in essence, the alpha and omega of the supervisory job. It is a beginning point in moving toward improvements in the way things are done, and it is a way of providing a closing appraisal designed to discern the outcomes of planned change.

Assessment is a powerful information tool for effective, innovative supervisors committed to the task of taking their people to where they have not been, in the interest of newness. It is a tool that rests on the skill of asking the right question at the right time, at the right place, and of the right people. Add to this skill the enthusiasm of the supervisory manager to take the initiative in posing questions, seeing the importance of asking the right questions, and giving these questions the priority they deserve. As Henry Ford once stated,

Health Care Superv, 1987, 5(2), 1–10
© 1987 Aspen Publishers, Inc.

"Enthusiasm is at the bottom of all progress. With it, there is accomplishment. Without it, there are only alibis."

The total act of assessment, in fact, goes beyond the single phase of appraisal, since the final payoff of engaging in evaluation is acting on what has been discovered. This point is made on the letterhead of policy letters sent out periodically to the managing directors of the Allied Stores Corporation:

> To *look* is one thing.
> To *see* what you look at is another.
> To *understand* what you see is a third.
> To *learn* from what you understand is still something else.
> But to *act* on what you learn is all that really matters.

As children, all of us knew quite intuitively, and quite well, how to ask questions. We endlessly sought answers. There is a classic story about a youngster who went riding on a New York City bus with his father. As they passed the Guggenheim Museum, the boy yelled out, "What's that, Dad?" "Don't bother me, son," was his father's reply, "I'm trying to read." During the bus trip downtown, the boy's spirit of curiosity at the sight of Rockefeller Plaza and the Empire State Building was again met with the same response from his father: "Can't you see I'm busy reading?" Finally, the little fellow said, "Gee, Dad, I hope you're not angry at me for asking so many questions." To this, his father replied, "Of course not, son. How else are you going to learn?"

The question "Why?"—the most potent query of them all—is the favorite of most youngsters. Eleanor Roosevelt referred to it as "a wonderful word that children, all children use. When they stop using it, the reason too often is that no one bothered to answer them. No one fostered and cultivated the child's innate sense of the adventure of life."

As we grow older and wiser, most of us leave behind the quality of the child—that of asking the question "Why?" along with "What?" "Where?" "When?" "Who?" and "How?" As adults, either we do not relish the idea of displaying any ignorance by asking too many queries, or we believe we already know most of the answers. Even if, perchance, we were to know all the answers, now all the questions are new!

In any event, what is required of today's supervisor, like all other levels of management, is to relearn the skill of inquiry. This can best be done by habitually exercising one's question-asking proficiency over time. The importance of sharpening the skill is underscored by the fact that the modern supervisor's task is not only one of answer giver, often viewed as the central task, but more significantly it is that of question asker.

To move the work unit from ordinary to extraordinary performance, the inquisitive supervisor must pull out all stops as a visionary so that the total system of conditions and circumstances is observed and challenged. After all, this is in keeping with a principal requirement of an ef-

The modern supervisor's task is not only one of answer giver, often viewed as the central task, but more significantly it is that of question asker.

fective manager, which embraces two interrelated thoughts: (1) understanding not only the organization's role in the health care system, but also the social, political, economic, and educational forces that affect the operation of the health care system, and (2) viewing the organization itself as a system in which all the components must interact and interrelate in order to effectively direct the hospital's resources to the treatment of the patient.

In line with these notions, four hierarchical levels of assessment are suggested that today's supervisor needs to engage in:

1. external assessment;
2. organizational assessment;
3. functional assessment; and
4. individual assessment.

Within each of these levels, clusters of questions are classified to further ensure the coverage of all subsegments of the system.

The intent here is not to offer an all-inclusive series of questions that should be posed by the supervisor at all four levels of assessment. Rather, it is to present a general pattern of thinking and inquiry that will assist supervisory personnel in formulating their own inventory of queries suitable to their own knowledge and re-sponsibility and to the situations and circumstances present within their existing environment.

EXTERNAL ASSESSMENT

To deal effectively with the complexities of the changing world of work, supervisors, like other managers within an organization, must extend their sights beyond the narrow limits of the functional boundaries of their own work units, even beyond the walls of the corporate system of which they are a part. They not only need to possess a sensitivity to the external forces affecting the operations of their hospital, they also need to be conscious of certain happenings in the outside world that may have a specific bearing on their operational activities. The larger system of which the organization is a part is a widespread territory that supervisors generally do not come in contact with, but it is important that they do so more and more if tomorrow's challenges are to be taken with increasing success.

With an eye on the outside world, the major focus that forms the subsegments within the external assessment activity would include the economic, demographic, social, political, and technical areas.

Under the *social* sector, for example, the supervisor should ask these kinds of questions relating to human resources:

- Are there any changes in individual value systems that might be expected in the period ahead?
- What new skills will be needed

in managing change and resolving people conflicts?

- In what ways will anticipated legislative decisions affect hospital personnel practices?
- What new professions will be on the health care scene as a result of new technology?
- Are serious shortages in certain areas of specialization being forecasted?
- Will union-organizing efforts tend to increase and be more successful in the future?
- In what ways will management skills become more essential in contract environments?
- What are the chances of increased financial pressures being a reality in the near future, and what effect will they have on the human resources of the organization?
- Are there to be changes in the industry that will affect education, retraining, and careers?

ORGANIZATIONAL ASSESSMENT

"A glaring misconception on the part of a majority of health care managers today is in viewing the hospital not as a *system* with interacting components, but as an organization composed of separate entities acting independently."[1] Indeed, all too many supervisors are independently "doing their own thing" without relating their efforts to the total organizational system. Their isolated actions are contrary to the well-established and

Today's supervisors constantly need to be engaged in assessing the status of their work units' interactions and interrelations with other components and processes of the hospital.

creditable principle that no single change is either good or bad until its effect on the total system is understood.

To further the value of seeing the organization as a whole, today's supervisors constantly need to be engaged in assessing the status of their work units' interactions and interrelations with other components and processes of the hospital. There are several divisions of questioning that should be embraced by the assessment, including:

- organizational goal setting;
- performance management;
- management process and practices;
- communication and coordination;
- quality improvement;
- financial administration;
- human resource management;
- training and education; and
- innovation and change.

Add to these categories of inquiry the organizational *processes* that specifically relate to the work unit for which the questioning supervisor holds managerial responsibility. A few examples of such processes are financial management, facilities and environment management, service program management, materiel management, and information systems management.

Using the above classifications as the assessment's structural form, consider a few selected questions that would appear to be proper within two of these focus areas. For example, under *performance management*, questions such as these might be included:

- Are organizational arrangements and support systems appropriate for attaining high levels of performance?
- Are expectations of supervisory performance clearly articulated throughout the organization?
- Are roles and responsibilities of the supervisor appropriately assigned and communicated?
- Is decision making sufficiently delegated down to the supervisory level of leadership?
- Are supervisors assigned proper scope and level of accountability?
- Does the administration's perception of performance hold to a good balance of its quantitative and qualitative dimensions?
- Are performance appraisals of supervisory personnel conducted annually? Have supervisors been appraised on an annual basis?
- Are the criteria upon which supervisors are appraised fair, sufficient, and objective?
- Is sufficient time and attention devoted to the performance evaluation discussion at appraisal

time and periodically throughout the year?
- Are supervisors adequately trained for the tasks they are required to perform?

Under the category of *communication and coordination,* questions such as the following would appear to be appropriate.

- Does the organization hold to the belief that obtaining information is an employee's right rather than a privilege?
- Are organizational communication channels open and free of "noise"?
- Are organizational policies, rules, and regulations clearly and adequately communicated?
- Is information throughout the organization accessible for current decision making?
- Does information flow freely up, down, and across the organization?
- Is goal sharing between and among functional areas a characteristic of the organization?
- Are supervisors provided with the information they need to fulfill their responsibilities?
- Do supervisory personnel in different operational areas have ample opportunity to interact and discuss common problems?

FUNCTIONAL ASSESSMENT

Once again, as with the previous higher levels of concern, the questions within the boundaries of the functional inquiry are not intended to be all-inclusive. Their purpose is to provide direction in employing an organized and analytical approach to improvement. Surely, the inquiring supervisor should go much further than the questions suggested.

Moving into the departmental, or functional, assessment phase, two kinds of questions are involved: first, the general type of questions that are considered appropriate for challenging work activities in all functional areas of the hospital, and second, the additional questions designed to address the particular uniqueness of any single department, primarily in terms of the nature of the work performed. These latter questions will be found most helpful as supplemental queries to the more general questions in use.

The classification of questions enveloped by the functional assessment provides the following kinds of focus categories:

- organizational purposes and direction;
- output analysis;
- input analysis;
- in-process analysis (work methods and procedures);
- personnel utilization and effectiveness;
- financial resources;
- materiel and equipment;
- information handling; and
- physical facilities.

Within the framework of two of the above divisions of questioning—personnel utilization and effectiveness and financial resources—the following list is a sampling of queries that would seem proper to ask so as to provide a beginning guide for supervisors in taking on the task of completing the remainder of their departmental or functional assessment tool.

Personnel utilization and effectiveness

- Is the structure of the department appropriate for the fulfillment of its mission?
- Are reporting relationships within the department satisfactory?
- Has the personnel complement of the department remained stable over the past three years?
- Are tasks being performed by the right persons?
- Are employees receiving adequate orientation and on-the-job training?
- Are the needed levels of skills in balance so that the best use is being made of the scarce skills?
- Are suitable replacements available if scarce skills are lost?
- Are regularly scheduled meetings being held with departmental employees?
- Is the upward flow of employee ideas being encouraged?

Financial resources

- Are costs reasonable in terms of the department's workload?
- Have operating costs remained at reasonable levels over the past few years?
- Are actual expenses within the limits of budget projections?

- Is money going into the right functions?
- Is there a reasonable relationship of overtime to sickness, vacations, and holidays?
- Has an estimate of cost by major types of work or procedure been developed for the department?
- Are employees in the department cost conscious and alert to possible cost control measures and approaches?
- Have employees been encouraged to give their suggestions for improving the efficiency of the department?

INDIVIDUAL ASSESSMENT

At this level of inquiry, the objective is to probe the opportunities for advancing the performance effectiveness of oneself as a supervisor, as well as the performance improvement of one's subordinates. It would seem reasonable to recommend the basic elements of the management process, namely, planning, organizing, communicating, motivating, and controlling, as the structural divisions of inquiry within the format of the individual assessment. Under motivating, for example, it is believed that these kinds of questions ought to be asked:

Motivating—for the supervisor
- Do I find my supervisory job to be challenging?
- Do I consider my work to be meaningful?

- Am I enthusiastic about the kind of work I do?
- Am I successful in establishing a climate of trust and confidence?
- Do I fairly and equitably apply personnel policies?
- Do I openly and frequently praise my people for doing good work?
- Do I effectively utilize participative management techniques and approaches?
- Are my own levels of competence in the fundamental areas of managerial performance such that they establish a good model for my employees to follow?
- Do I have in place a personal development plan?

Motivating—for the employee
- Are all of the employees reporting to me performing at levels of expectation?
- Do each of my employees exhibit a team attitude?
- Do employees respond in positive ways to growth opportunities?
- Are employees enthusiastic about their involvement in participative management efforts?
- Are there adequate indications that all employees have a high morale level and a willingness to perform?
- Do all employees evidence quality in their performance and conduct?
- Has there been an absence of employee grievances and complaints over the past 12 months?

- Are all departmental employees adequately trained for the job they perform?

THE BENEFITS OF ASSESSMENT

It is the question that awakens the mind; but it is the action taken to solve the identified deficiency that provides the ultimate benefits. And there are many benefits to be realized. They come in two varieties: (1) those that are measurable, and (2) those that are intangible, or unmeasurable. The latter type is quite important, for if such benefits are not sought after and achieved, it is possible that significant measurable benefits may not be forthcoming.

Measurable benefits include
- dollar savings;
- labor savings;
- productivity improvement;
- quality enhancement;
- increasing innovation;
- greater operational efficiency;
- improved communication and coordination;
- supervisory skill building and role change;
- progress in employee participation;
- reduction of expensive waste; and
- more problems solved, and at the right level.

Intangible benefits include
- stimulation of organizationwide improvement activity;
- improvement in delivery of care and service;
- utilization of human talents to a greater extent;
- improvement of employee morale and job satisfaction; and
- accommodation of creative people.

SOME PRINCIPLES AND PRACTICES

To move toward the realization of these kinds of benefits, it is essential for the questioning supervisor to take note of certain recommended principles and practices of inquiry. Here are some of the more significant ones to keep in mind as the assessment process is put to work.
- Since there are no perfect solutions there is always room for improvement.
- It is not only the act of gaining new knowledge that is essential, it also is necessary that the disposition to crave knowledge is always present—the *want* to know.

In pursuing the inquisitive process, there should always be an overriding concern about the questions that are not asked.

- In pursuing the inquisitive process, there should always be an overriding concern about the questions that are *not* asked.
- Above all, the questioner needs to be an optimist.
- In experiencing self-assessment, it is important to find value in

knowing what is being experienced.

- The advice of David Lloyd George should be heeded. "Don't be afraid to take a big step if one is indicated. You can't cross a chasm in two small jumps."
- While there is the need to uncover facts, they should not be allowed to get in the way of imagination.
- Listening is the key to questioning. Listen closely for quality questions, and listen carefully to the responsive words as the words are actually uttered.
- The habit of saying yes to a new idea needs to be formed, and the words of Charles F. Kettering need to be recalled: "If you have always done it that way, it is probably wrong."
- By asking questions, problems are shared with others, which is the first step in solving any problem.
- In the process of self-assessment there is always a place for spontaneity—that quality of trusting one's own instincts.
- Be wary of the appeal of the one preferred solution selected in the absence of tracking down other possibilities. As H.L. Mencken once advised, "For every problem there is one solution which is simple, neat and wrong."
- There are no shortcuts in the essential tasks of appraising and evaluating. In keeping with this principle, we are reminded by the classic saying that "a shortcut is often the quickest way to some place you weren't going."
- It is important to remember that the objective of assessment is to ask questions that are problem directed, not solution directed. The latter comes into play after a problem is identified and there is the need to move toward a desirable resolution.
- The cry of "I don't have time" is a faulty claim, since a value of assessing is that it will most often result in gaining additional time for the questioning supervisor and his or her people.
- Self-assessment is everyone's business, and when the supervisor initially sets the direction and pace, employees will follow with ease. Why? Because the act of questioning is contagious.
- Self-assessment holds little regard for assumptions, for the chances are that those in supervisory leadership positions do not ever really know as much as they think they know or as much as they should know about the way in which things are being done in their areas of responsibility. Supervisors can test this proposition by simply assessing something that is assumed to be working well and then be a witness to the breaking apart of the assumption as the right kinds of questions are applied with patience and perseverance.
- Good questions tend to lead to better questions. Thus, "piggy-

backing" is a helpful game to play when self-assessing.

- "Men are never so likely to settle a question rightly as when they discuss it freely" (Southey's Colloquies, 1830).
- What is required is a systems vision of reality on the part of the inquisitor, who needs to be aware of the essential interrelatedness and interdependence of all that is being questioned. Thus, whenever possible, questions posed at the different levels of assessment should be designed to have a relationship with each other. (It will be noted that there is a relationship among the examples of communication questions appearing at the three levels of organizational, functional, and personal assessment.)
- A central purpose of assessment is to create new conditions and circumstances. A saying of George Bernard Shaw comes to mind: "People are always blaming their circumstances for what they are. I do not believe in circumstances. The people who get on in this world are the people who get up and look for the circumstances they want, and if they cannot find them, make them."
- There are two common characteristics of ineffective inquisitors: They are superficial observers, and they do not always want to hear the answers.
- What is essential is intelligent questioning if assessment is to work. Intelligent questioning means having a concern for the individual being questioned and for the human factors contained in the surrounding environment.
- There is some truth in Voltaire's familiar saying, "Judge a man by his questions rather than by his answers." Surely, the strength of a good supervisory manager lies in his or her ability to ask the right questions where there is an absence of understanding, and to ask these questions with an open mind, with an absence of any preconceived notions. Indeed, for the supervisor in any operational area of the hospital, the question mark is a mark of distinction.

For Isador Isaac Rabi, one of this nation's greatest physicists, inquisitiveness was certainly his mark of distinction. Having grown up as a boy in lower Manhattan, he recalls his mother asking him each day as he returned from school, "Isador, did you ask any good questions today?" Surely, a question that all supervisors should ask themselves at the close of each working day is "Did I ask any good questions today?"

REFERENCE

1. Bennett, A.C. *Improving Management Performance in Health Care Institutions.* Chicago: American Hospital Association, 1978, p. 105.

Is productivity coming into its own— Again?

Charles R. McConnell, M.B.A., C.M.
Vice President for Employee Affairs
The Genesee Hospital
Rochester, New York

A ONE-PAGE advertisement for a publication dealing with the topic of productivity landed on many health care managers' desks. This ad claimed: *The most pressing problem you face today is how to meet your community's growing health care needs with shrinking resources.* The advertisement and accompanying sample publication had much more to say about the necessity of improving productivity, of doing more with less in the delivery of health services.

Another source advises us: "Continual improvements within the hospital are necessary, not only because of the worthiness of hospital goals, but because of the economic impact of hospitals upon all people, collectively and individually. The magnitude of this impact may be seen by examining the economics of hospital facilities, operation, and utilization in the United States."[1]

The foregoing passages sound much like the legitimate concerns of today, as those who operate health care organizations

Health Care Superv, 1992, 10(3), 75–85
©1992 Aspen Publishers, Inc.

struggle to make each dollar work harder, while others, both internal and external to health care, to try to slow the growth of health care costs. The fact of the matter is, however, that these concerns were voiced more than a quarter century apart; the advertisement appeared in 1991 while the second passage was written in about 1965. Health care productivity, it would seem, has been a concern for some time.

But has the concern for health care productivity been consistent? And have efforts been applied to improve productivity?

FAD AND PRACTICE

Similar to the likes of motivation, commitment, and quality, productivity is a concept-in-a-single-word that is misused more frequently than it is constructively applied. Productivity is one of the different-shaped gimmicks in the management tool box that every once in a while is pulled out and polished up and examined in a supposedly new light.

In health care, productivity became a magic word during the latter half of the 1960s. During the 1960s health care costs began to climb dramatically, fueled by the mid-decade establishment of Medicare and Medicaid along with advancing technology and ever-intensifying modes of treatment. Productivity improvement quickly became much of health care's supposed cure for many of its own ills. The challenge of productivity improvement soon became a challenge of measurement; if the results of a particular human activity were to be improved, there would have to be a means available for measuring those results both before and after the improvement intervention. In short, the apparent need was for measures of output.

There was a great deal of activity with measures of output—so-called "standards"—during the latter half of the 1960s and into the 1970s. Much of the activity was grant funded, supported at least in part by government, foundations, and various not-for-profit organizations such as state and regional hospital associations. All based in some way on the work measurement techniques of industrial engineering, various approaches included:

- the "Michigan Methodologies," a series of manuals developed at the University of Michigan consisting of detailed predetermined time standards applying to various hospital operations, including separate manuals for a number of clinical and support activities;
- the "CASH-LPC" (Commission on Administrative Services to Hospitals-Labor Performance Control), a California development, like the Michigan methodologies a compilation of predetermined time standards and time-standard "building blocks" from which one could synthesize standards for similar activities;
- the work of various hospital management engineering programs, including programs of the Hospital Association of New York State (HANYS), Massachusetts Hospital Association (MHA), Chicago Hospital Council, New Jersey Hospital Association, Ohio Hospital Association, and a number of other programs.

Hospital management engineering came into its own—supposedly. No more than industrial engineering under another name, due primarily to the ready resistance within health care to anything "industrial," management engineering emerged in two forms: inhouse engineering and shared management engineering services.

Some hospitals employed their own management engineers and even established management engineering departments. Many other hospitals participated, through membership in various associations, in the establishment of shared management engineering programs. These programs were often established as fee-for-service adjuncts of hospital associations, that is, an association service that was paid for not by the general membership through dues but by only the actual users of the service. In effect this put a number of association engineering programs in the management consulting business.

Cost escalation and the matter of productivity were of sufficient importance in the 1960s that steps were taken to encourage the formation of shared management engineering programs that would operate on a not-for-profit basis. Foundation grants were provided to start a number of programs under the auspices of various hospital associations. Other grants went to fund the development of productivity measurements in the manner previously described.

Once started, management engineering programs proliferated dramatically. Before the decade of the 1960s ended, one early cooperative effort, the Western New York Hospital Management Engineering Program, had become the source of people who went on to establish several other regional programs in New York State and several statewide and multi-state programs in other

---

Once started, management engineering programs proliferated dramatically.

---

parts of the country. For a few years these programs recruited capable industrial engineers from manufacturing and from engineering schools and kept them productively occupied.

For a few years productivity was "in." For a few years productivity was a broad-spectrum cure for the apparent ills of the health care industry. However, the rocket of productivity that flew into fashion starting in the middle 1960s had all but sputtered out by the middle 1970s.

THE FAD BOWS TO LONG-TERM EFFECTS

By 1975, through mergers and dissolutions, the number of active hospital management engineering programs throughout the country had fallen significantly, and many surviving programs found their staffing and activity levels greatly reduced. Productivity improvement was no longer trumpeted as a universal solution. By 1975, in fact, some programs were turning away from promoting improvement through management engineering and turning toward improving hospitals' operating results through reimbursement rate appeals and otherwise "gaming" the growing number of reimbursement regulations to ensure maximum reimbursement under the prevailing system.

A number of factors and forces seem to have come together in varying degrees to dull the glow of hospital productivity improvement by the mid-1970s:

- *The productivity honeymoon ended.* As far as health care was concerned, "productivity" was one of the fad words and hot concepts of management during part of the '60s and '70s. In health care as well as in all other lines of endeavor, the historical path of management is littered with fads and hot concepts that had their day and either fell by the wayside or settled into a useful existence on some modest or minimal scale. We find, along the way at various times, management by objectives, Theory X and Theory Y, matrix management, Japanese management, as well as productivity. (In the 1990s the emerging hot concepts for health organizations surely include guest relations and continuous quality improvement or total quality management.) The honeymoon period with any "new" approach inevitably ends for two reasons: Much of the commitment to the fad of the day is shallow, lip-service commitment, and as soon as the glow of the fad begins to fade, the commitment is withdrawn; the hot concept, as valuable as it may prove to be over time, is invariably shown by time to be far less of a cure-all than it was first thought to be.

- *External funding ended.* As mentioned previously, a number of shared management engineering ventures were started with grant funding. Arrangements were such that, for example, a foundation put up half of the money to start a program, with the remainder coming from the institutions that used the service. However, most grant arrangements were, understandably, time limited; they expired after a while (three years was a fairly common grant timeframe), after which the service was expected to be self-sustaining through user fees. Given many commitments to productivity improvement that were not particularly strong or long standing, many using institutions fell away as

costs increased and the bargain nature of the service dissipated.
- *Competition arose.* As start-up funding gradually ran its course and user fees increased, management engineering programs found themselves in the management consulting business in direct competition with commercial consulting firms. As the costs of the not-for-profit programs approached those of the for-profit consultants who also benefitted from name recognition, some service users found they had other options. Essentially the shrinking productivity improvement market was being carved up by an increasing number of providers as management engineering programs became redefined as members of the management consulting industry.
- *Much of the easy work had been accomplished.* In its first few years of activity in hospitals, management engineering accomplished a great deal. Some sound, high-dollar savings were generated. And it made a great deal of sense to promote management engineering by tackling the most visible savings opportunities and showing some impressive returns. However, as the easier tasks were accomplished and the projects became more difficult, it became necessary to dedicate more time and resources to undertakings for which the likely returns were neither impressive nor especially apparent. Once again, as the road became tougher, superficial commitments dissipated.
- *There were negative effects of productivity improvement.* Some health care institutions suffered financially to an inordinate degree because they had

cared enough to save money. As a few of the states adopted cost-based reimbursement programs in which a hospital's income would be based on its costs in some earlier year plus an inflation adder, it became apparent that an efficient hospital would receive less payment for the same service than an inefficient hospital. Some payment systems encouraged inefficient hospitals to remain that way (until acted upon by other forces, namely newer and different regulations) and discouraged others from becoming more efficient because doing so appeared to exact a direct financial penalty.

- *Internal management engineering involves visible cost.* Management engineering in a hospital is a staff function; it is clearly not a patient care function. Like other staff functions it exists to support the organization's line functions in their delivery of patient care. Management engineering is also not a revenue-producing activity, and under the pressure of reimbursement regulation it has been necessary to look closely at all activities that entail costs without producing revenue. Although management engineering exists in large part to produce savings—such a function should regularly save its own costs and then some—the returns on this activity are not always readily apparent. Once the easy, visible savings have been realized, much of the management engineering task becomes one of maintenance—of keeping the lid on creeping overstaffing, for example, and monitoring numerous activities for cost increases while still looking for ways to be more productive. It is extremely dif-

ficult to accurately and completely determine the savings impact of a mature management engineering function. However, it is simple to reckon the cost of that function, and as a staff function it is frequently a target for reduction when hard times impact the bottom line. The fate of the productivity improvement function then hinges on the relative visibility of various costs: the single amount of money required to operate the function (its budget) is easy to see, but the dollars that will drift through cracks and crevices without the function are for all practical purposes invisible.

- *Politics, politics, politics.* Productivity improvement requires measurement and productivity measurement requires standards. Obtaining standards requires that values, usually in terms of time which of course translates into money, be placed on most human activities in the organization. Here the standard reactions to so-called "industrial" approaches come into play: we simply cannot measure certain activities ("We're not building automobiles, you know; *we* deal in human life") and the generally erroneous but deeply held belief that it is not possible to reduce costs without adversely affecting quality. There are few if any human activities that cannot be placed "on standard," but variable, complex activities performed by largely self-determining technical and professional employees—that is, much of a hospital's work—are far more difficult and expensive to measure than repetitive manufacturing activities. And the standards created for such activities are subject to sufficient variation that they can always be challenged by someone who does not wish to be held to them. In addition there are the interdepartmental political considerations of an organization that traditionally tends toward being a collection of semi-autonomous operating entities and the problems presented by medical staff, mostly nonemployees who by virtue of their status wield considerable power and authority within the organization. Also, one might insert at this point everything that can be said about addressing resistance to change.

THE GOVERNMENT SPEAKS UP

It was not health care alone that saw productivity improvement as an urgent need from the mid-1960s to the mid-1970s. In the late 1960s much was made of apparently declining national productivity, to the extent that in 1970 a National Commission on Productivity and Work Quality was established. The commission comprised seven major committees, one of which was the Hospital and Health Care Committee made up of nearly 75 people from about 20 health-related organizations. Issued in 1975, the Hospital and Health Care Committee's report made a number of recommendations.[2] The following comments highlight the report's 10 primary recommendations and briefly describe what might have occurred concerning each in the more than 15 years since the report was issued.

1. *Development of a reimbursement system with built-in incentives to include comprehensive coverage for ambulatory care services.* Marked progress has been made in this area since 1975. The pressures of reimbursement are diverting more and more ac-

tivity to the outpatient side, and although positive incentives to use outpatient care are increasing, much has been forced by the negative incentives associated with the continued use of inpatient services.

2. *Expanded implementation and continued evaluation of health maintenance organizations (HMOs) and other comprehensive fee-paid health plans.* Such approaches were seen in 1975 as offering options to the public and physicians alike while taking advantage of economies of scale. Progress has been significant in this area, with HMOs and related alternatives such as preferred provider organizations (PPOs) steadily growing in numbers. In some parts of the country the penetration of such options now stands at more than 50 percent.

3. *Increased use of management engineering services and techniques, preferably through statewide shared services programs.* As was the case in 1975, only about one-fourth of hospitals have management engineering services. The committee recommended sharing of such services because many hospitals were seen as not large enough to economically operate their own services. However, the number of statewide and regional shared management engineering programs has decreased since 1975, and management engineering studies aimed at improving productivity are presently far fewer than during the productivity heyday of the late 1960s and early 1970s.

4. *Promotion of the formation of multiinstitutional mergers such as those in*

As was the case in 1975, only about one-fourth of hospitals have management engineering services.

the investor-owned and religious sectors of the health care industry. The greatest numbers of merged institutions remain those that are part of proprietary and religious chains. However, a noticeable number of nonprofit community hospitals are merging into larger systems, although a number of mergers have come about as a last alternative short of closure. Recent signs suggest that short of merger there is considerable room to be explored for looser ties between institutions, arrangements that might be called affiliations or working agreements that permit some economies of scales while preserving each participating hospital's independence.

5. *Expansion of shared services programs by hospitals.* Sharing of certain nondirect services, for example purchasing and laundry services, remains active and healthy as in 1975. Additional services, such as waste disposal, are finding their way into the shared service arena. There is still not a great deal of sharing in evidence in clinical or direct care areas.

6. *Development and expansion of hospital employee incentive programs.* Bonus and incentive programs for upper management personnel have been gradually but steadily spreading throughout the industry. Incentive programs that involve all employee levels have been still slower in catching on. There remain some legal barriers, in that certain nonprofit institutions can place their tax-exempt status at risk by paying bonuses. Also, in the highly regulated states the issue of incentive or bonus payment frequently withers in the presence of a negative operating line.

7. *Continuing education programs for middle management personnel in health care facilities.* This is today as much of a need as it was in 1975. If anything, today's need for continuing management education is far more acute than previously. In addition to productivity issues and other issues that remain, with recent years' proliferation of laws affecting employment, we are now faced with dramatically increased needs for management education about discrimination and employee rights.

8. *Expansion of the role of the hospital administrator in the policymaking of the institution.* Little appears to have changed since 1975; relatively few administrators are voting board members.

9. *Expansion of the role of the business sector of the nation's economy in the delivery of health care.* The committee rightly pointed out that business is a large purchaser of health care and suggested that business needs to learn more about health care and use its expertise to help improve health care productivity. In recent years business has clearly become more interested and involved, but not in the way the committee envisioned. Business has been reacting, with a clear sense of urgency that sometimes seems to approach panic, to the dramatically increasing cost of health care insurance coverage. The company that increases its employees' share of the health insurance premium or increases the employees' deductibles and copayments is not trying to improve health care productivity; it is trying to control its health care costs, period. The business reaction to increasing costs also increases the pressure on third party payors to force economies within the health care system by limiting reimbursement increases. Business involvement will continue to grow in the foreseeable future, but much will remain focused on how to limit businesses' health insurance premium costs.

10. *Increased involvement and/or responsibility of physicians in both the general and*

financial management of health care institutions. A relatively small proportion of short term, nongovernmental hospitals have physicians on their governing boards; this was also the case at the time of the committee's report. Since physicians prescribe care and services and generally influence hospital expenditures heavily, they should be both involved and accountable. There may be problems working out the kind and extent of physician involvement, but there is little doubt about the need to involve them.

The foregoing suggests a fairly mixed collection of responses to the committee's recommendations of 1975, but overall not much has happened in terms of impact on health care productivity. That there was little follow-up at all to the committee's report might suggest that the problems of shallow commitment were fairly widespread.

WHY BE CONCERNED ABOUT PRODUCTIVITY?

It is reasonable to ask why we should be concerned about productivity, especially in the face of reimbursement systems that only indirectly encourage concern for productivity. Productivity deserves attention because:
- it is simply good management to want to apply available resources to best effect;
- it is possible, in an organization as varied and complex as a modern hospital, to redistribute resources from areas of savings to other essentials;
- the inflationary spiral affects all business entities, and when resource inputs grow at a rate faster than system outputs, the costs to the consumer increase;
- we should wish to maintain a voluntary system, and to do so the costs of health care cannot continue to rise out of pro-

portion to all other sectors of the economy;
- there is increasing external pressure to hold costs down while continuing to produce quality health care.

Further, concern about productivity needs to be ongoing. One of the common errors of productivity's heyday was to regard productivity improvement as a one-time effort that could sweep through an organization and make it more efficient for all time. Not so. Some of the larger, more obvious corrections are one-time changes, but the need for attention to productivity is continuing. Left unto itself, an activity will be subject to creeping inefficiencies that eventually accrue to a significant problem. Creeping inefficiencies are the drift that will eventually take the raft up against the shore as it moves with the current; constant attention to operating efficiency is the pressure on the tiller that maintains the raft in the channel. Left unto themselves, most human activities will suffer diminished productivity; regular attention is needed to keep them tuned and running efficiently.

COMING INTO FAVOR ONCE AGAIN

It was mentioned earlier that the National Commission on Productivity and Work Quality came into being in 1970 because American productivity had declined in the late 1960s and had yet to show signs of recovering. Productivity statistics appar-

Some of the larger, more obvious corrections are one-time changes, but the need for attention to productivity is continuing.

ently indicated some degree of gradual recovery through the 1970s; many people probably assumed the problem had gone away. There are, however, more recent indications that the problem has returned, if indeed it has ever been too far away at all.

A July 1991 news story from the Associated Press carried the headline, "U.S. Standard of Living Falls for First Time Since '82."[3] The story reported that Americans' standard of living declined slightly in 1990 "as the country fell further behind in its ability to compete internationally,"[3(p.9A)] according to the Council on Competitiveness. Specifically: "The council said in its fourth annual competitiveness index that America lost ground in such key areas as living standards, productivity, and investment."[3(p.9A)]

The council's index measures the relative performance of the world's seven richest industrial countries. According to the report, the U.S. was the only country to experience an outright drop in living standards last year, and for three consecutive years had ranked last of the seven in terms of the share of its economy devoted to investment.

The Council on Competitiveness is, of course, dealing primarily with manufacturing concerns, but the references to living standard, productivity, and investment relate to the entire American economy. With health care accounting for a significant portion of our gross national product, there is no denying the impact of health care on our national statistics.

In addition to signs from the economy at large such as the foregoing, there are other indications suggesting that productivity is now or is soon to be "in" again. Although much of the concern over runaway cost inflation in health care will be reflected in the direct efforts of some businesses and third party payors to simply pay less, there will inevitably be renewed close examination of operations for potential improvements in productivity. If an institution is to have to do more with the same resources or do the same with less, it follows that responsible management will seek all reasonable ways of improving productivity.

Another current force that is bringing productivity back into prominence is the current interest in quality as evinced in the concept of total quality management (TQM) or continuous quality improvement (CQI). The quality issue is inextricable from the productivity issue; one has direct implications for the other, and there is a direct relationship between quality and productivity (one decidedly different from the misconception cited early in this article, that productivity gains are made only at the expense of quality).

Although coming again to the foreground, productivity will probably not this time around be limited to the perceived methods-improvement, cost-cutting, staff reduction activities frequently associated with management engineering. Although work measurement may play a large part in productivity improvement, the view of productivity and thus the scope of future effort will likely be more global than past efforts.

PRODUCTIVITY IN SIMPLEST TERMS

In any activity productivity is represented by a relationship between input and output; that is:

$$output/input = productivity$$

Any process or activity has associated with it a level of quality, describing quality as the relative acceptability of the output. Any change in productivity involves changes between and among all of these factors. That is, productivity may be said to be improved if:

- output is increased while input is held constant or decreased and quality is held constant (doing more with the same or less);
- input is decreased while output is held constant or increased while equality is held constant (doing the same or more with less);
- quality is improved while input and output are held constant or reduced (doing better with the same or less).

It follows, then, that productivity is reduced if the opposite of any of the foregoing changes occurs, for example, if output should decrease while input is held constant.

This simple concept begins to complicate rapidly when the need for measurement is introduced. It is in obtaining and using measures of productivity that myriad personnel and political problems occur and that significant expenses can accrue. However, whether one uses gross productivity guidelines such as average expected nursing hours per patient day, or specific, activity-related time standards, such as 1.5 minutes (0.025 hr.) to fill out a maintenance work requisition, there will have to be some expression of output per some unit of time for most human activities in the organization. There can be a great deal of work involved in obtaining these expressions, but recall the productivity improvement spurt of the 1960s and 1970s—and appreciate that much of the work of provid-

ing the means for building standards has already been done.

IT NEVER LEFT

Productivity may have cycled in and out a time or two depending on the superficial fad aura that has occasionally attached to it, but the concept of productivity and the need for constant attention to it has always been with us. The overall objective of productivity improvement efforts will remain the enhancement of the accomplishment of work by doing things in less time or with less effort or at lower cost while maintaining or improving quality.

The principal factors influencing productivity are:

- capital investment;
- technological change;
- economies of scale;
- knowledge and skill of the work force; and
- work methods, procedures, and systems.

These factors should also be recognizable as encompassing most of the basic needs of enterprise. While the control of capital and technology and scale economies might reside largely with top management or the governing body, there remains much that the individual supervisor or middle manager can do to improve productivity. By working continually to increase the knowledge and skill of the work force, by being constantly aware of the need to improve work methods, procedures, and systems, the conscientious supervisor or middle manager can make continuous productivity improvement a fact of working life.

REFERENCES

1. Smalley, H.E., and Freeman, J.R. *Hospital Industrial Engineering.* New York, N.Y.: Reinhold Publishing Corporation, 1966.
2. National Commission on Productivity and Work Quality. *Report of the Hospital and Health Care Committee.* Washington, D.C.: Government Printing Office, 1975.
3. *Democrat and Chronicle,* Rochester, New York, 10 July 1991, p. 9A.

Performance auditing for health care supervisors

Robin E. Scott MacStravic
Vice President
Planning and Marketing
Health and Hospital Services
Bellevue, Washington

PERFORMANCE auditing is a systematic, quantitative process that "audits" or assesses the performance of individual departments based on selected criteria. Its purpose is to identify how successful a department is at a given moment. Performance auditing is intended to be of primary value to the department supervisor as the basis for planning, evaluating and managing departmental activities.

Performance auditing fulfills three purposes for health care supervisors. First, it provides a systematic description of how well a given department is doing at any point in time. Second, it provides the basis for setting standards, goals and objectives that can be used to manage activities on an ongoing basis and achieve significant improvements in operations. Third, it provides the basis for making important decisions that would

Health Care Superv, 1984,2(2),67–77
© 1984 Aspen Publishers, Inc.

either alter or perpetuate the way the department functions.

There are three major areas of a department's operation that are assessed in a performance audit. First, there is the financial area: how successful is the department in terms of costs standards, revenue generation, conformance to budget? Second is the operational area: how efficiently and effectively is the department performing its function and contributing to the organization as a whole? Third is the marketing area: to what extent is the department satisfying its public, the other department's employees, physicians or patients it serves?

SUCCESS CRITERIA

The key to effective performance auditing is the identification of clear and explicit success criteria. In order to know how well things are going, the right "things" must be specified and then examined. The things that should be examined are whatever most clearly and completely capture the values of the organization and each of its contributing parts. For a given department, success criteria should reflect what makes its internal functioning good or bad, plus what makes its contribution to the organization good or bad.

Internal criteria

Every department has success criteria that reflect its internal effectiveness. Its ability to operate within budget, its productivity or efficiency,

its professional standards of quality, etc., are examples of internal success criteria. Such criteria are used by those working in a department to judge their own performance. They are used as quality control standards to keep internal operations on target and within acceptable norms.

Such internal success criteria would typically include the following categories.

- *financial performance*—costs per unit, rate of increase per year, labor costs, equipment costs and space and supply costs compared with industry norms (Hospital Administrative Services [HAS] cost comparisons are examples of financial performance indicators.);
- *service*—units of service provided, such as admissions processed by admissions department, bills processed through billing and collections, X-ray films, laboratory tests, square footage of floors cleaned, meals served (this is a measure of how much of the department's or program's major function was accomplished);
- *quality*—quality of service provided using whatever measures and standards are appropriate (e.g., accuracy of laboratory tests, cleanliness of rooms, completeness of medical records per the Joint Commission on Accreditation of Hospitals [JCAH], etc.);
- *resources*—the quantity and quality of resources available compared with standards or

ideals (number of personnel slots filled, proportion of certified technicians, status of equipment, adequacy of space, supplies, etc.);
* *efficiency*—the amount and quality of service provided for the resources used, productivity of personnel and equipment, overall output provided for input expended;
* *satisfaction*—of employees in the department, measured by numbers of complaints, formal survey ratings, absenteeism, turnover, union activities and other indicators.

Internal measures

To use the above success criteria effectively each must be translated into objective, measurable indicators that can be regularly monitored, reported and understood.

Financial measures:
* actual expenditures to date compared with budget;
* percent increase in budget from last year to this year;
* specific costs for space, supplies, labor, etc., compared with other organizations of similar size and scope of operation; and
* revenue generated versus last year, versus budget.

Service measures:
* actual numbers of services rendered in all areas; and
* rate of increase in service compared with increase in organization's overall business activity.

Quality measures:
* proportion of laboratory tests found to be accurate when checked by an outside laboratory;
* proportion of medicines provided accurately and on time by nursing staff;
* nutritional quality and appearance of meals served; and
* proportion of rooms passing inspection.

Resources measures:
* proportion of personnel slots filled;
* proportion of workers satisfying certification criteria where applicable;
* square feet of space as percentage of recommended need; and
* proportion of time equipment is fully operational versus down.

Efficiency measures:
* nursing and other full-time equivalents per patient day; and
* personnel time per unit of service.

Satisfaction measures:
* turnover, absenteeism and tardiness rates; and
* job satisfaction ratings of employees.

Measuring internal performance requires the use of some quantifiable dimension of the department's activity that can be measured accurately and cheaply, plus a basis for comparison. There should be a measure for every value of importance to the department or program. Normally such values will fall into one of the foregoing categories, but if a value is impor-

> *Measuring internal performance requires the use of some quantifiable dimension of the department's activity that can be measured accurately and cheaply.*

tant it should be measured even if it does not fit in the above list. In addition, there must be some basis for interpreting the results of measurement. Industry norms, professional standards or the organization's own perceptions may be used. The important notion is to be able to determine when the department's performance according to a measure is unacceptable, acceptable, admirable or anywhere in between.

External criteria

In addition to internal performance measures reflecting what people think about themselves, each department or program serves what is essentially an external market. Everyone not working in the department or program but nevertheless affected by it is part of the external market. To at least some extent, internal department performance measures should reflect how successful the department is in serving such markets. In general, external success criteria will fall into one or more of the following categories.

- *Image*—how the department is viewed by other departments or programs in the organization, by

physicians, by patients and the community, by peers, and by competitors. The department's reputation will have much to do with how well it fares at budget time and with what the organization's overall reputation will be.
- *Use*—how much the people who have a choice use the department's services compared with how much they use other alternatives, and what share of potential business the department actually enjoys.
- *Contribution*—what demonstrable impact the department has on the organization's overall performance, as reflected in the performance audit, and by the extent to which the department's contribution is recognized and appreciated (relates to *image*).
- *Satisfaction*—the extent to which people doing business with the department—the other departments and programs that relate to it—have their expectations satisfied by the department's services.

In contrast to internal success criteria and measures, these external criteria reflect more the *consequences* of what the department does and how it accomplishes its purpose. Moreover, these are largely subjective measures involving people's perceptions and attitudes, rather than objective data that may be a matter of record. The single objective criterion, namely utilization, is a specific market-success criterion and directly reflects subjective preference.

External measures

Because they are mainly subjective, external success criteria are harder to measure and often require explicit survey efforts to find out how a particular department is perceived by others. How often a department tries to find out how it is perceived should be a function of how important these perceptions are and whether the department is trying to alter them. Chances are the department should be devoting more time and effort to such perceptions than it has in the past.

Some examples of specific, external success measures that might be used are

Image measures:
- proportion of people (other employees, patients, physicians, community) rating the department as the best in town or very good to excellent on some rating scale; and
- proportion of people elsewhere in the organization who know what the department does, where it is located and how it contributes to the organization's overall success.

Utilization measures:
- proportion of employees eating in the cafeteria, for example, or other hospitals using a shared laundry service—everyone who has a choice but who chooses to do business with the department in preference to anyone else.

Contribution measures:
- identifiable improvements in the organization's financial health,

image, service, quality, use, efficiency, resources, contribution and satisfaction that are attributable to the department's efforts; and
- proportion of employees and physicians who credit the department with achieving that contribution.

Satisfaction measures:
- scaled ratings of the department's services by other departments, patients, physicians or family as appropriate; and
- numbers of complaints versus praises received in person or in writing from other departments, patients, physicians, family, etc.

DEVELOPING APPROPRIATE CRITERIA

Because a department's success criteria will reflect both internal and external success values, the selection of appropriate criteria and measures should be carried out with fairly wide participation. Employees of the department should participate because they will be evaluated based on the criteria selected. Representatives of other departments served or otherwise affected by the department should participate because they represent the department's external market. Such participation need not involve large numbers of people meeting together, since groups larger than six or eight are likely to be ineffective. Small groups can be used to identify specific types of criteria and measures.

One exception to this pragmatic approach is that at some point the department's employees and representatives of the markets they serve should discuss together the types of values that should be included in the performance audit. Often by acquainting employees with the impact their efforts have on the rest of the organization, a stronger identification with the organization as a whole can be built and a greater sensitivity to the department's importance can be developed.

Including representatives of other departments should also assist when the time comes to take actions aimed at improving the department's performance. There should always be links between improving the department's success and improving the success of other departments. Identifying the impact of proposed changes on the rest of the organization should facilitate getting budgets approved where proposed changes require significant new expenditures. If the value of the department can be explicitly identified, it should have better luck in budget discussions even where no significant changes are proposed.

MEASURING PERFORMANCE

Once the appropriate categories of performance criteria and a useful set of success measures have been developed, performance auditing moves to collecting information. The data needed to identify where the department stands on any specific measure may be derived from one or more of the following sources: (1) existing records, (2) surveys and (3) observation.

Existing records of the organization should provide most of the financial data, service information, quality and resource measures required. Data on efficiency of the department's use of resources and indirect measures of employee satisfaction should also be available in personnel and operational records. Some effort may be required to refine such data down to the departmental level, but normally this will be a relatively simple process.

Surveys will be required for any and all measures addressing the perceptions and attitudes of people. The only way to discover the department's "image" in the organization is to ask a representative sample of people whose image of the department is of concern. Satisfaction of those di-

---

The only way to discover the department's "image" in the organization is to ask a representative sample of people whose image of the department is of concern.

---

rectly served by the department will also have to be assessed via survey. In addition, some aspects of utilization choices can be ascertained only by asking people: when they have had a choice, what portion of the time did they seek the department's services as opposed to going elsewhere? The contribution made by the department may be demonstrable through systematic records, but the extent to which that contribution is recognized can be determined only by asking people.

There are a variety of approaches that can be used in determining people's perceptions and attitudes. If the number of a specific group of people of interest to the department is relatively small (e.g., physicians), individual discussions may be arranged on a relatively casual basis. Where numbers are larger, a sample may be drawn in some representative fashion. Invite a sample of people whose opinions the department cares about to discuss their perceptions over coffee or lunch.

For some publics (e.g., patients at large) a formal questionnaire survey may be advisable. Where numbers are very large, and the possibility exists that people might be reluctant to share their true opinions, such a survey may be the best approach. An outside organization should probably be used to ensure that the data collected are both statistically valid and unbiased. Such surveys are expensive but may be used to measure perceptions regarding all departments, thereby reducing the cost of information to each.

The informal approach can be effective not only in gathering data but in communicating to groups of people the department cares about. The very fact that representatives of the department seek out such people communicates interest and concern. Asking for comments regarding satisfaction, image, utilization choices and contribution suggests a willingness to respond to the problems or distresses of others. Care should be taken to respond to concerns that are expressed, however, or else such contacts serve only as gripe sessions and may increase dissatisfaction levels.

Observation should always be included among data collection techniques. Walking through the work area is a good way to assess activity levels and morale in addition to relying on records or surveys. The supervisor who frequently observes the activity of each employee is communicating interest and may see correctable situations before they show up in records or complaints. Asking employees to observe each other on an occasional basis demonstrates respect for their opinions and can facilitate sharing of experiences, provided they do not turn into backbiting battles.

Whatever approach is taken to measuring performance, it should meet two requirements. First, it should actually measure what is supposed to be measured. Turnover rates may not truly measure employee satisfaction, for example, if a downturn in the local economy keeps everyone in his or her job, regardless. Second, and related to the first, is that everyone who participates in the performance audit should accept the measure as both valid and significant. Otherwise the audit process becomes a meaningless exercise.

Using the audit

Once a number of appropriate and manageable success criteria and measures have been identified, they can be used in any or all of the following ways.

1. *Assessing present performance:* The success of the department, how well it is doing at any point in time, can be assessed in terms of explicit, measurable values. The fact that its relations with the public and with other departments within the organization are included gives everyone a basis for evaluating how well it is doing.

2. *Targeting improvements in performance:* The assessment of present success should result in identification of specific success measures that should be improved (problems), that might suffer decline unless acted on (threats) or that can be significantly improved (opportunities). Any targeted change in success that requires new or extra effort serves as an objective to justify such effort and as a basis for selecting the most effective type of effort to apply.

3. *Evaluating efforts:* Any proposed change in the department's operations, regardless of who proposes it, should be evaluated in terms of the foreseeable impacts on explicit success criteria. Unless the proposed change represents significant promise of improved success, is worth the cost and is the best promise available, it should not

be implemented. Once implemented, the change should be monitored and evaluated in terms of what its actual effects have been.

Table 1 suggests specific criteria, measures and sources of data for two illustrative departments: a specific nursing unit and the housekeeping department. These are suggested as illustrations more than recommendations for such departments, but supervisors may find one or more of them useful.

Cautions

The use of explicit success criteria employing objective measures of departmental performance is not without risks or problems. Many of the potential difficulties of this process have been encountered in attempts to implement management by objectives (MBO). The chief hurdle encountered in using explicit success measures is the reluctance of people to be judged by factors not totally within their control. This is an almost universal human trait, and it is one that must be dealt with carefully in performance auditing.

Many of the department's success measures, especially those of the internal type, will be familiar and unthreatening to employees. The external success measures, however, may be both unfamiliar and threatening. Employees may feel uncomfortable at the thought of being held accountable for what other people think of them (image), how successful they are in competitive situations (use) or

Table 1. Specific criteria, measures and sources of data for nursing and housekeeping

| Criterion | Nursing | | Housekeeping | |
	Measure	Data source	Measure	Data source
Financial	Expenditures compared with budget	Budget records	Expenditures compared with budget	Budget records
Services	Patient days of care rendered	Utilization records	Number of rooms cleaned	Department records, logs
Quality	Percent of charts meeting nursing audit standards	Nursing audit records	Number of rooms meeting inspection	Inspection records
Resources	Percent of slots covered by shift Mix of RNs, LPNs, aides	Personnel/payroll records	Complaint rate, e.g., number per 100 patients	Correspondence or complaint reports
Efficiency	Nursing hours per patient day	Payroll and utilization records	Percent of slots covered Absenteeism levels	Personnel records
Image	Physician rating of quality Numbers of nurses waiting to be hired or transferred to department	Survey of physicians Personnel records	Housekeeping hours per patient day	Payroll and utilization records
Utilization	Percent of beds filled compared with other units	Utilization records	Community and physician ratings of housekeeping, cleanliness, appearance	Survey
Contribution	Ratings by other departments	Survey	Cleaning nearby physicians' offices	Department records
Satisfaction	Patient ratings of care received	Survey	Rate of increase in costs compared with other departments Nursing, patient and family ratings of cleanliness	Budget records Survey

how satisfied other departments are with their efforts (satisfaction).

There are two key approaches to reducing employee concerns about the use of external success criteria. The first is to ensure that employees realize the importance of external success measures, in terms of both organizational success and their own personal values. The budgetary benefits of good external performance should be emphasized. The second key is to introduce external objectives gradually. Assuming that there are a number of external success measures that could stand some improvement based on the first performance audit, let the employees themselves choose which to work on and how best to do so.

Because the use of explicit success measures and the accountability it involves are threatening, this approach should be introduced gradually with careful selection of initial targets or objectives. One of the biggest problems with MBO has been the tendency to set objectives for everything. Objectives should be set regarding only significant performance values for which significant change is required to achieve significant improvement. Standards may be employed to guide efforts aimed at maintaining current performance. If objectives are set on routine values for which no changes are required or no real improvement is expected, they become numbers games.

The vast majority of success measures examined in a performance audit should be found to be acceptable just as they are. Employees should be praised for their positive achievements in all such cases. Only a few criteria and measures should be targeted for improvement at any one time. This avoids giving employees the feeling that they are always going to be expected to work harder and produce more year after year after year.

Initial targets for improvement should be chosen carefully, with full participation of the employees who must change or intensify their efforts to achieve improvement. The amount

> *The amount of improvement targeted should be achievable rather than ideal, and should be of significant value to the employees themselves as well as to the organization.*

of improvement targeted should be achievable rather than ideal, and should be of significant value to the employees themselves as well as to the organization. The best type of targets are those that are: (1) achievable within a short time—no more than a year; (2) clearly visible when achieved, therefore sure to be noticed by the employees and organization; and (3) significant to the organization's success criteria and to the success of specific other departments.

By selecting initial targets carefully and working to ensure their achievement, the supervisor accomplishes two important results. First, the department will be noticed for promising and then delivering a significant improvement in its and the organization's success. Second, the employees of the department will be introduced to performance auditing in a rewarding and nonthreatening manner.

As employees accept and become enthusiastic about using explicit success measures, they are likely to begin targeting greater and greater improvement. While their enthusiasm should be maintained, their optimism should be guarded. The supervisor should ensure that promised improvements are nearly always delivered in full. This means using careful judgment about what sort of promises to make. Most success measures should probably be maintained at present acceptable levels rather than targeted for improvement on a regular basis. Those measures for which change is targeted should be modest in number but significant in value and highly likely to be accomplished.

These outcome criteria should not become devices for pressuring employees toward ever-receding objectives, however. Employees themselves should participate in determining which performance measures should be improved and how. The supervisor must be open to suggestions by employees as to how improvements can be accomplished. Rewards should be provided for *maintaining* good performance on most criteria as well as for improving performance on a few, when possible. Where performance is improved through department-wide effort, the entire department should be rewarded.

EXPECTED OUTCOMES

The use of explicit success criteria in regular, systematic performance auditing should produce significant outcomes for the department supervisor. First, it should provide a basis for an effective assessment of where the department stands, how successful it is and how valuable it is to the organization. Second, it should sensitize employees to the significance of their efforts in terms of explicit organizational values. Third, it should provide a meaningful basis for reward and recognition of employees, both individually and collectively.

This approach to performance auditing must be used carefully, but it can produce significant benefits to the supervisor, the department and the organization. It will afford greatest benefit when the organization as a whole also engages in systematic performance auditing. As in any management technique, performance auditing should be learned and implemented carefully and used as a stimulus to positive effort rather than as punishment. By focusing the department's attention on explicit success values and directing the organization's attention to the department's contribution, performance auditing should result in greater recognition of the department as well as greater success for the organization.

SUGGESTED READINGS

Bennett, A. *Improving Management Performance in Health Care Institutions.* Chicago: American Hospital Association, 1978.

Deniston, O., Rosenstock, I., and Getting, V. "Evaluation of Program Effectiveness." *Public Health Reports* 83, no. 4 (1968): 323.

Levinson, H. "Appraisal of What Performance?" *Harvard Business Review* 54, no. 4 (1976): 30.

MacStravic, R. "Strategic Outcome Planning Promotes Goal-Oriented Hospital Management." *Hospital Progress* 64, no. 2 (1983): 42.

Meyer, H., Kay, E., and French, J. "Split Roles in Performance Appraisal." *Harvard Business Review* 43 (January–February 1965): 123.

Raia, A. "Goal Setting and Self Control." *Journal of Management Studies* 2, no. 1 (1965): 34.

Work smarter, not harder

Addison C. Bennett
Management Consultant
Los Angeles, California

IN 1982, the editors of *Fortune* authored the book *Working Smarter,* a theme originally expressed by Allan H. Mogensen a half century ago.[1] Mogensen, an industrial engineer working at Eastman Kodak in the 1930s came upon a discovery that changed the world of analysis and improvement of work. Then, as now, engineers, like Mogensen, whose arena of work was to study the output of others were called "efficiency experts" by people on the line who either resisted or resented the changes being proposed and implemented by these experts.

Mogensen's idea was not only innovative, but workable. It was simply this: to gain the acceptance of workers to change and to motivate them at the same time, to teach them some basic engineering approaches and to solicit their ideas for improving the way they do things so that they will not only "work smarter," not harder, but will also be recognized and rewarded for their suggestions. The name Mogensen gave to this

Health Care Superv, 1988, 6(3), 1–13
© 1988 Aspen Publishers, Inc.

approach was *work simplification*. This approach is based on the fundamental proposition that "the person doing the job knows far better than anyone else the best way of doing that job and therefore is the one person best fitted to improve it."[2]

The author, as a student of Mogensen, first introduced the philosophy and programming of work simplification in the retailing sector, and subsequently in the health care industry. In both situations, significant cost-effectiveness and high levels of job satisfaction were achieved as the result of employee participation in the search for work improvement.

In the early 1960s, management, or industrial, engineering arrived on the health care scene as a valued discipline. Two-and-a-half decades later, extensive attention is being given to professional engineering practices; yet, at the same time, there is little focus on the value and usability of involving people on the job as analyzers and improvers of work methods and procedures.

It is in error to view the application of engineering and work simplification as an either/or issue. Rather, they should be perceived to be complementary and supportive of each other so that the natural outcome is one in which cost, productivity, and quality problems are attacked most effectively and efficiently through a blending of the specific skills of the professional engineer with the job insight and detailed knowledge of the individual employees themselves, both at management and nonmanagement levels.

The concept of work simplification, which also may hold the identity of methods improvement or work study, is an idea whose time of arrival has been ignored too long. And it is one great way to get back to basics that offers high potential payoffs.

WHAT CAN THE SUPERVISOR DO?

In a discussion of work simplification, it would seem reasonable to follow an outline that adheres to one of the fundamental elements in the search for discovery, that is, the use of the following key questions: What? Where? When? Who? How? and the all-important Why?

Beginning with the *What* of improvement, two main questions come to mind: (1) What is the starting point for the supervisor? and (2) What can the supervisor do from that point on?

Becoming knowledgeable about work simplification is the first order of business and should include discussions with a management engineer and a course or texts covering the subject. Two books[3,4] written about the subject specifically for the health care industry can prove helpful to the innovative supervisor. With insight and understanding of principles, approaches, techniques, and methodologies, along with personal experiences in their applications, the interested supervisor can move ahead in his or her own area of responsibility. This forward movement can occur even in the absence of an ideal situation, that is, having a management engineer on staff or having an organization-wide cost-effectiveness/productivity effort under way.

Regardless of the performance qualities top management expects in its supervisors, one attribute will underlie all other qualities—the ability to be an effective problem solver. Obviously, this capability calls for the supervisor to have a positive attitude toward change and improvement, and thus an effective involvement as an agent of change. This involvement stems from three basic qualities:

1. *Curiosity and discontent.* An old maxim says that without discontent, curiosity becomes idle; with curiosity, discontent is only useless hand-wringing. The supervisor must avoid complacency. Walton expressed it this way:

   Complacency, the feeling that all's right with the world, especially with us, is a comfortable feeling. It is when we fear that this comfortable state of affairs may be upset that we go into action, or when it has been upset, we act to restore it. It is doubtful if we ever do anything at any time except to prevent our complacency from being disturbed and recover it if it has been disrupted.[5]

   The supervisor must regard all work habits and patterns with suspicion if his or her efforts to implement change are to be successful.

2. *Open-mindedness.* In the constant search for improvement, the health care supervisor must be open to new arguments and ideas. The supervisor must be free from decision making based on mental inflexibility and immovably fixed opinions. A lack of an objective receptiveness to the suggestions of others and a tendency to prefer his or her own ideas can seriously impair the supervisor's effectiveness in any problem-solving undertaking.

3. *Self-respect.* As an agent of change, the supervisor must respect his or her own ability to resolve problems relating to operational performance. The supervisor can take a big step forward by adopting the philosophy that an organized and systematic plan for achieving work improvement will be more helpful and more effective than a haphazard, trial-and-error approach.

APPLYING A SYSTEMATIC APPROACH

Beyond the day-to-day management of a department or work unit lies the requirement for systematic analysis and improvement, based on careful study of the department's objectives, procedures, problems, and resources.

To carry out a problem-solving process designed with thoroughness and regularity, the improvement-minded supervisor should follow these steps: recognize, examine, and evaluate the problem before installing a new plan to solve the problem.

Recognize

Recognition includes identification, selection, and definition of the problem situation. During this first step, the supervisor attempts to develop a complete list of work situations that may offer improvement possibilities, and then establish an order of priority for the various work problems that have been identified.

The following questions can be helpful to the supervisor in setting study priorities:

- Which problem situation is causing the most difficulty?
- How soon must a solution be found?
- Is the problem situation really the one to be solved, or is it simply a part of a still larger problem?
- Is the timing for the study appropriate from the standpoint of employee turnover, absenteeism, work demands, and personalities involved in the job situation?

- Is there a good chance of achieving improvement?
- How soon can discernible results be attained? What will the extent and the nature of the benefits be?
- How long has it been since changes were introduced in the job in question? What happened?
- What are the attitudes of personnel toward the existing process or procedure? Is employee resistance or resentment anticipated?

Examine

Examination includes the collection and analysis of all relevant facts surrounding the existing problem situation and the development of possible alternative solutions.

There are various ways of gathering facts about any work problem. Among the most effective ways are the supervisor's own observations of the situation; interviews and discussions with personnel concerned with, or involved in, the problem; reference to existing records; and the accumulation of current data by operating personnel.

Regardless of the performance qualities top management expects in its supervisors, one attribute will underlie all other qualities—the ability to be an effective problem solver.

It is important for the supervisor to remember that the successful assembling and analyzing of data will depend on the accuracy with which the information is recorded. Therefore, it is important to avoid relying on hearsay when collecting facts about the problem under investigation. Nor is memory reliable, since most people do forget details and too often remember a situation or a circumstance as they *want* to remember it rather than as it actually occurred.

In analyzing the facts that have been collected and recorded, the supervisor needs to apply a logical sequence of questions to all phases of the job activity:

- *What* is being done? Why is it being done? What else might be done?
- *Where* is it being done? Why is it done there? Does it need to be done at that particular place? Where else might it be done?
- *When* is it done? Why is it done then? Does it need to be done at that particular time? When else might it be done?
- *Who* is doing it? Why does that person do it? Could it be done better by someone else? Who else might do it?
- *How* is it being done? Why is it done that way? How else might it be done?

Evaluate

Evaluation of the various alternatives under consideration also includes reaching a decision about the best and most effective method available.

At this stage of the study, the supervisor evaluates each listed suggestion for improvement potential and selects those ideas that he or she feels should be made part of the improved method. The task of developing an improved method requires that five basic questions be answered:

1. What should be done?
2. Where should it be done?
3. When should it be done?
4. Who should do it?
5. How should it be done?

Any decisions made about these five questions must be in keeping with the initial statement of the problem situation and the study objectives. Moreover, the decisions should have been made with the advice and the assistance of individuals directly concerned with improving the existing method.

Install

Installation involves the planning, installation, and maintenance of the new and improved method. The importance of this last step is not to be underestimated. Certainly as important as any of the three previous stages of the problem-solving procedure, it is perhaps the most difficult of all.

PRINCIPLES

In all four steps is a set of principles of thought and behavior essential to furthering the supervisor's capability for change and his or her ability to effect change. These principles include the following:

- *Innovation* involves wondering afresh, thinking creatively, and breaking with routine.
- *Perspective* concerns the problem solver's manner of viewing things, and his or her attitude. (Finding a way out of a problem calls for optimism and humor.)
- *Humanism* values thought, attitude, and behavior concerned with human beings and their interests and welfare.
- *Participation* relies on the help of others to solve a problem and to gain acceptance of and support for change.
- *Perseverance* calls for continuing strength or patience in dealing with problem situations.

- *Objectivity* shuns the influences of emotion, surmise, or personal prejudice.
- *Measurement* puts to rest the problem-solving bugaboos of "I think," "I guess," and "I'm not sure."
- *Inquiry* calls for an open mind and the absence of any preconceived notions.
- *Wholeness* underscores the need to view and approach problems in their totality.

VALUABLE TECHNIQUES

As facts about the existing method are collected, they should be recorded to facilitate their subsequent analysis. Fortunately, the data compiled in connection with many problem-solving situations can be presented graphically in charts or diagrams, making the analysis easier and much more productive. The benefits of charting techniques include the ability to

- more effectively analyze and improve work activities,
- present information in a clear and concise manner,
- save many hours of study activities,
- help in "selling" recommended changes to the employees—and to the boss, and
- use excellent training aids in teaching new methods to employees.

In terms of technique, one analytical tool is simple to use, has a wide range of application, and has proved highly effective in the examination stage. That tool is the Flow Process Chart, an excellent technique for determining how the step-by-step details of a job are actually being performed. The chart provides a simple means of recording a series of events, start to finish, within a particular procedure or work activity. If a printed Flow Process Chart is not available, an 8-1/2 inch by 11 inch lined sheet of paper with a hand drawn grid will suffice.

The Flow Process Chart, like a motion picture camera, places each step of a method or procedure in its proper frame of sequential order and in a documented form. Following the recording of this motion picture of facts, the analytical supervisor can examine and evaluate these documented events until discoveries emerge.

Giving testimony to the value of work simplification and flow charting, Andrew S. Grove, president of Intel, said:

Automation is certainly one way to improve the leverage of all types of work. Having machines to help them, human beings can create more output. But in both widget manufacturing and administrative work, something else can also increase the productivity of the black box. This is called *work simplification*. To get leverage this way, you first need to create a flow chart of the production process as it exists. Every single step must be shown on it; no step should be omitted in order to pretty things up on paper. Second, count the number of steps in the flow chart so that you know how many you started with. Third, set a rough target for reduction of the number of steps. In the first round of work simplification, our experience shows that you can reasonably expect a 30 to 50 percent reduction.[6]

A significant reduction can be achieved in the number of steps required to perform almost any task. Take, for example, differences between the present and proposed flow of work on a nursing floor as displayed in Figures 1 and 2.[7] While simple in context, this example of improvement does point up vividly the kinds of opportunities that may lie within an organization, waiting for someone to bring about an improvement. When added to many other increments of change, these opportunities can ultimately result in significantly greater effectiveness and efficiency.

Like other techniques of analysis, the Flow Process Chart naturally has its constraints. It is vertical in its nature of recording, thus excluding the benefits of viewing the problem situation in its more dynamic form. To do this, the supervisor turns to a related graphic tool, the Flow Diagram, that clearly shows the movement of the subject being examined, as well as the layout of the work area (see Figures 3 and 4).[8]

The value of the Flow Diagram lies in its capability to display graphically the paths of movement of people, paperwork, or materials in order to visualize the whole process. This capability is particularly desirable in work situations in which the distance traveled is excessive, the flow is complicated, the work area is congested, or backtracking is evidenced.

The Flow Process Chart, like a motion picture camera, places each step of a method or procedure in its proper frame of sequential order and in a documented form.

The creativity of the supervisor plays a role in developing flow diagrams for more complicated problems. For example, various line patterns such as lightly and heavily drawn lines, dots, or broken lines, can be introduced. Also different colors can be utilized to simplify the reading and interpreting of the diagram.

The vertical nature of the Flow Process Chart, while ideal for gathering and record-

FLOW PROCESS CHART

PAGE *1* OF *1*

SUMMARY

		PRESENT		PROPOSED		DIFFERENCE	
		NO.	TIME	NO.	TIME	NO.	TIME
○	OPERATIONS	7					
⇨	TRANSPORTATIONS	5					
□	INSPECTIONS	1					
D	DELAYS	3					
▽	STORAGES	2					
	DISTANCE TRAVELLED	75 FT.		FT.		FT.	

JOB *USE OF MEDICATION CARDS ON NURSING FLOOR*

☐ MAN OR ☐ MATERIAL _____
CHART BEGINS *IN CARD BOX*
CHART ENDS *IN CARD BOX*
CHARTED BY _____ DATE *6/12/62*

	DETAILS OF (PRESENT/PROPOSED) METHOD	SYMBOLS	DISTANCE IN FEET	QUANTITY	TIME SEC.	ANALYSIS WHY?	NOTES	ACTION
1	MEDICATION CARD IN MEDICATION CARD BOX	○⇨□D▽					LOCATED IN TRAY ROOM	
2	CARD TAKEN FROM BOX	○⇨□D▽					OCCURS APPROXIMATELY 50 TIMES EACH DAY ON EACH FLOOR	
3	CARRIED TO NURSES' DESK	○⇨□D▽	25		15			
4	CHECKED WITH KARDEX	○⇨□D▽			30			
5	CARRIED TO MEDICINE CABINET	○⇨□D▽	25		15			
6	PLACED ON TRAY	○⇨□D▽						
7	WAITS WHILE MEDS ARE POURED	○⇨□D▽						
8	CARRIED TO BEDSIDE WITH MEDS	○⇨□D▽	VARIES					
9	WAITS WHILE MEDS ARE GIVEN	○⇨□D▽						
10	PLACED IN NURSES POCKET	○⇨□D▽						
11	CARRIED BACK TO DESK	○⇨□D▽	VARIES					
12	REMOVED FROM POCKET	○⇨□D▽						
13	PLACED ON DESK	○⇨□D▽						
14	WAITS WHILE MEDS ARE CHARTED	○⇨□D▽			45			
15	PICKED UP FROM DESK	○⇨□D▽						
16	CARRIED TO MED. CARD BOX	○⇨□D▽	25		15			
17	PLACED IN MED. CARD BOX	○⇨□D▽					Located in Tray Room	
18	REMAINS IN MED. CARD BOX UNTIL NEXT MED IS GIVEN	○⇨□D▽						

Figure 1. Flow Process Chart showing present method of using medication cards on the nursing floor. Reprinted with permission from Preston Publishing Company, New York, New York.

ing facts relating to a single item process, is not particularly adaptable to more complex work procedures. When used in presenting the details of a rather lengthy and involved activity, the chart becomes unwieldy and difficult to follow. For this reason, it may be necessary for the supervisor to use an alternative route—a Horizontal Chart.

Unlike the Flow Process Chart, which reflects the job in a single vertical column,

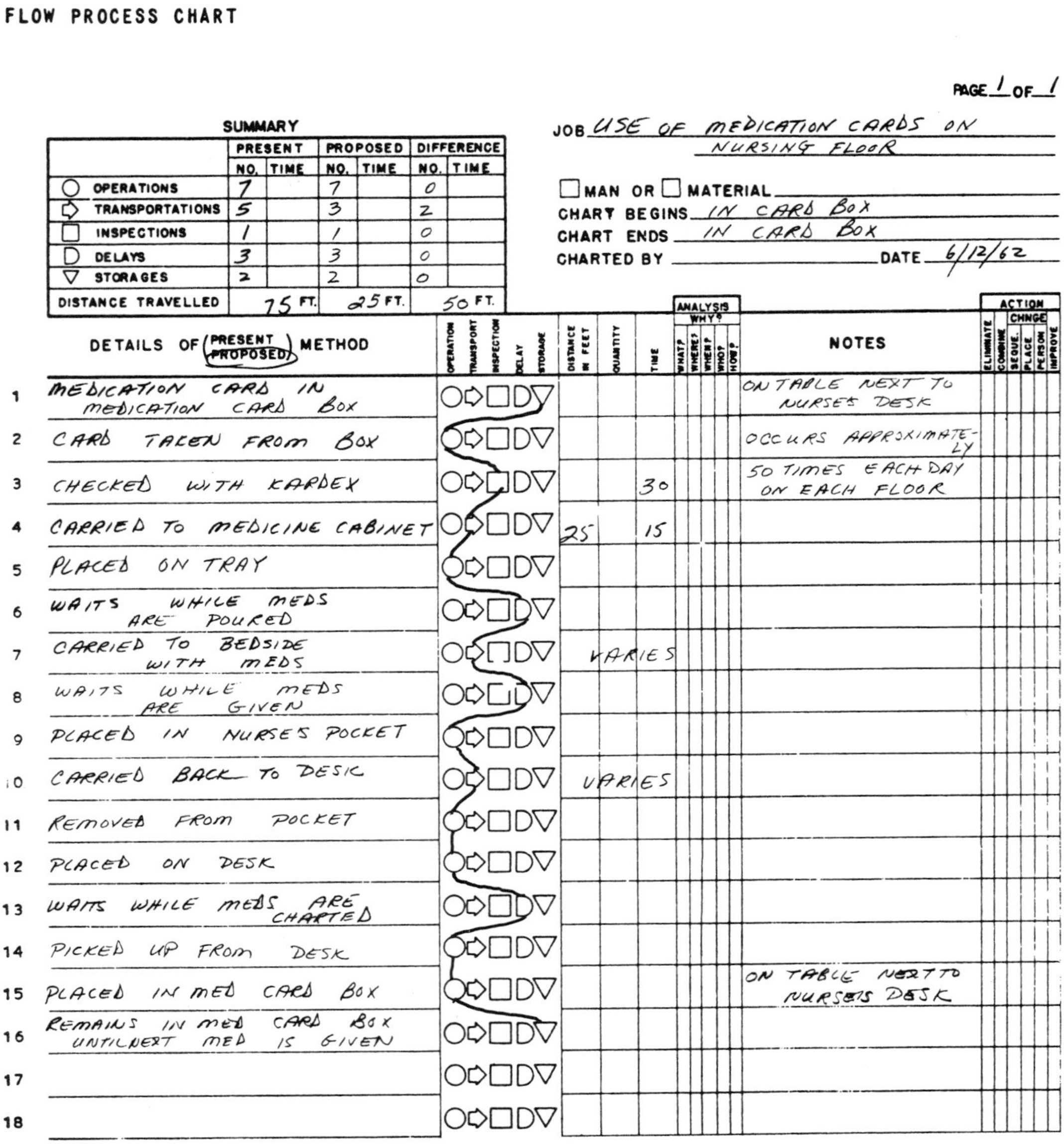

FLOW PROCESS CHART

Figure 2. Flow Process Chart showing proposed method of using medication cards on the nursing floor. Reprinted with permission from Preston Publishing Company, New York, New York.

the Horizontal Chart is a multicolumn form that captures the descriptive words and symbols in a left-to-right sequence.

The use of the Horizontal Chart is recommended when the procedure being studied involves the performance of many different work routines by individuals in different departments. It also may be used for recording the step-by-step details of procedures that involve printed forms with more than one part or more than one copy (see Figures 5 and 6).[9]

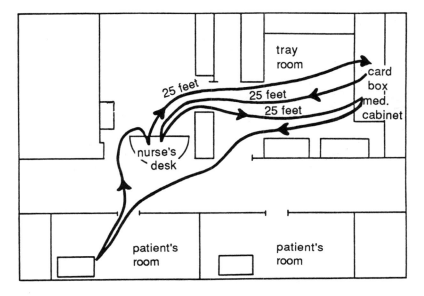

Figure 3. Flow Diagram showing present method of using medication cards on the nursing floor. Reprinted with permission from Preston Publishing Company, New York, New York.

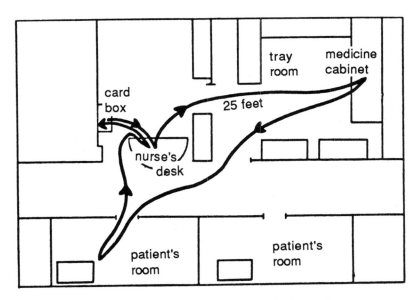

Figure 4. Flow Diagram showing proposed method of using medication cards on the nursing floor. Reprinted with permission from Preston Publishing Company, New York, New York.

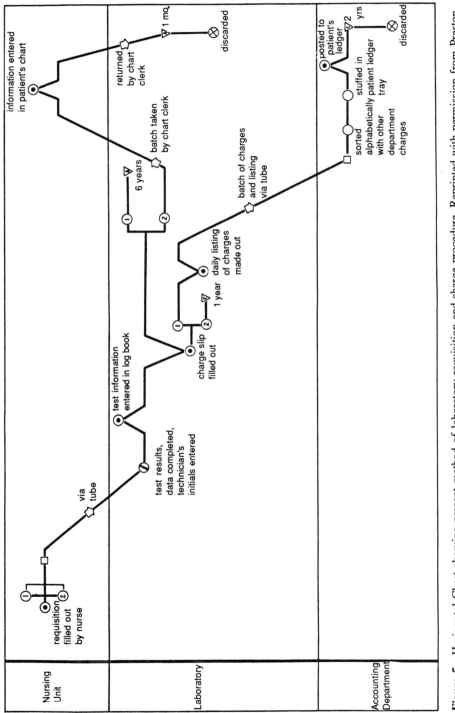
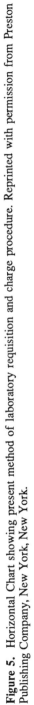

Figure 5. Horizontal Chart showing present method of laboratory requisition and charge procedure. Reprinted with permission from Preston Publishing Company, New York, New York.

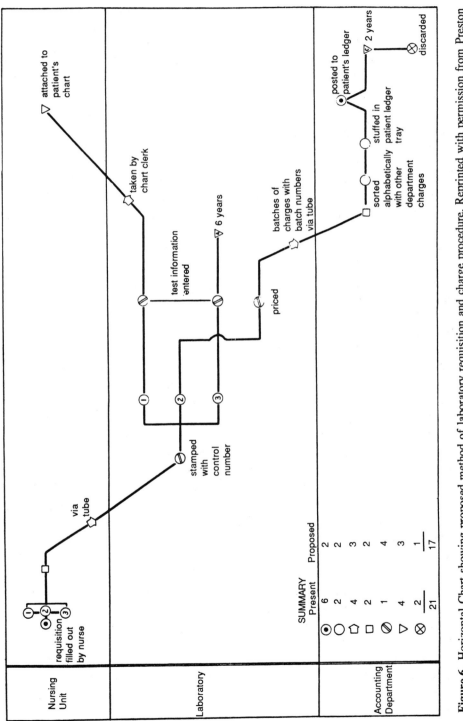

Figure 6. Horizontal Chart showing proposed method of laboratory requisition and charge procedure. Reprinted with permission from Preston Publishing Company, New York, New York.

APPLICATIONS

Where can these approaches and techniques be applied? In just about any corner of the enterprise where work is performed. In addition to work activities that relate to care, comfort, and service to patients, six other areas offer improvement potential:

1. *Administration*—management functions such as planning, reporting, directing, and scheduling.
2. *Clerical operations*—office functions such as sorting, checking, recording, and filing.
3. *Communications*—presentation and transmission of verbal or written messages from one point to another.
4. *Transportation*—system or mode of conveyance of persons or materials from place to place.
5. *Utilization*—method or manner in which personnel, space, or materials are used.
6. *Loss or accident prevention*—performance control and safety functions to prevent loss or injury.

The change-minded supervisor's sensitivity to the presence of indicators or "signals" can be helpful when zeroing in on specific areas of improvement potential. Examples of signals that frequently indicate the presence of a problem include:

- backlog of unfinished work in any operation;
- delays and interruptions in the performance of a function or service;
- overtime that is needed repeatedly to carry out an activity;
- waste of effort, equipment, material, personnel, time, or space;
- complaints from patients, personnel, or visitors;
- unduly high costs of the function;
- continual absenteeism or turnover in any organizational area;
- loss or damage of supplies or equipment, and injury to employees and others;
- congestion or disorderliness in a work area involving one or more individuals;
- excessive time devoted to an activity in proportion to the actual end result;
- location of an object in an out-of-the-way place; and
- fatigue due to walking, bending, reaching, or other nonproductive or tiresome work motions.

CONTINUING SEARCH

There is only one response to the question, "*When* should the search for improvement occur?" and that is, "On a *continuing* basis, of course." The response is the endless retort, "I'd do it, if I could only find the time." Chances are slim in today's hurried world in which most people are performing assigned tasks that any individual will find the time demanded by the search for a better way. What is required is that the individual *make* time. Interestingly, one sure way of gaining the luxury of "loosening up" the constraints of time is to find ways to save time through effective problem-solving practices and techniques capable of eliminating, combining, or simplifying elements of work previously thought to be immutable.

Who needs to be part of the continuing search? All members of the organizational family do, since improvement for the sake of cost-effectiveness, productivity enhancement, and quality advancement is everyone's business.

If including all employees within the work simplification framework is an acceptable idea, we are then led to the final questions: "*How* do we involve them?" and "Why?"

Central to the participative effort is the supervisor's teaching and training role. This role requires the leadership qualities of excellence, sharing, unity, and innovativeness—all of which employees can witness as the supervisor brings subordinates together in a continuing series of educational sessions designed to move the work group to superlative levels of performance, promote interaction and exchange of ideas, create togetherness and harmony, and bring newness and novelty to the workplace through the solicitation and implementation of employee ideas for improvement.

The basic objectives of the inservice educational process should be directed toward providing employees with the following:

- a thorough understanding of the history of the organization's progress in improving patient care and service, and of the importance of change in organizational growth and progress;
- insight and recognition of certain obstacles to effecting changes for improvement;
- an awareness of the significance of achieving improvements in a systematic manner; and

- an indoctrination in the problem-solving techniques that will assist them in developing ideas for improvement.

To achieve these objectives, the supervisor needs to prepare an adequate oral presentation, and should plan to distribute written and illustrative material to participating employees. The supervisor also should consider using visual aids such as slides, posters, and charts.

●　　●　　●

Both the supervisor and his or her employees benefit from the continuing participative process. The supervisory manager experiences a greater sense of self-satisfaction as increasing influence over the destiny of his or her own area of responsibility is exercised. The nonmanagement employees, too, hold good feelings about being engaged in meaningful work.

For the majority of people in today's work force, the idea of meaningful work contains two ingredients: (1) the opportunity to identify problems that lie in the way of doing a good job, and (2) positive encouragement to be a part of the improvement process that leads to the solution of these problems. Indeed, work simplification serves both of these purposes well.

REFERENCES

1. Editors of *Fortune. Working Smarter.* New York: Viking Press, 1982.
2. Ibid., viii.
3. Bennett, A.C. *Methods Improvement in Hospitals.* New York: Preston Publishing, 1975.
4. Bennett, A.C. *An Employee Idea Program for Hospitals and Nursing Home Type Facilities.* New York: Preston Publishing, 1974.
5. Walton, A. *New Techniques for Supervisors and Foremen.* New York: McGraw-Hill, 1940, p. 86.
6. Grove, A.S. *High Output Management.* New York: Random House, 1983, p. 35.
7. Bennett. *Methods Improvement in Hospitals,* 18, 31.
8. Ibid., 21, 31.
9. Ibid., 69-70.

Cost containment: a new way of life

Charles R. McConnell
Vice President for Employee Affairs
The Genesee Hospital
Rochester, New York

IT IS NO SECRET to people who work in health care or to those who deal with the health care industry as consumers that health care costs are increasing. Neither is it unknown to most persons that health care costs are rising significantly faster than most other costs of living and are consuming an ever-expanding share of the nation's total resources. The nation's population is enjoying generally better health and longer life than ever before and receiving better health care than has ever been available to the citizens of any country, but it is paying for these unquestioned benefits at a dramatically increasing rate.

STAGGERING STATISTICS

In 1960 total health care expenditures in the United States amounted to approximately 5½ percent of the

Health Care Superv, 1985,3(3),66–77
© 1985 Aspen Publishers, Inc.

GNP; by 1980 health care expenditures as a percentage of GNP had grown to approximately 9½ percent.[1] During the same 20 years, 1960 to 1980, total U.S. health care expenditures rose from about $30 billion to $250 billion per year. In other words, in 20 years the national health care bill multiplied more than eight times.[2] During the same 20-year period, hospital room rates increased by more than 600 percent and physicians' fees rose more than 300 percent.[3]

It is true that the total population of the United States increased markedly from 1960 to 1980. However, per capita health care expenditures have increased at a rate far outstripping the increase in the numbers of people. In 1960 per capita health care expenditures in the United States were $146.30; by 1980, annual health care expenditures had risen to an average of $1,067.06 for every man, woman and child in the United States.[4]

A disturbingly high level of health care cost is not simply a specter that might someday appear. It is already present in a number of dimensions. In late 1983 it was related by former Health, Education, and Welfare Secretary Joseph Califano that:

- Health care costs account for more than 10 percent of the GNP.
- Health care expenses exceed defense outlays as the fastest growing portion of the federal budget.
- Health care costs, not income taxes, are the biggest item in the gap between an employer's total compensation costs for an employee and the amount of pay that employee takes home.[5]

Health care costs in the United States are increasing at a rate roughly double the national rate of inflation. It is estimated that by 1990 the national health care bill will have reached $850 billion per year—on the average, $3,700 per year for every person living in the United States.[6]

A frequently asked question is: What are the causes of this seemingly runaway escalation of health care costs? Do they lie primarily in medical advances of such compounding sophistication that more complex skills, more exotic drugs and more expensive equipment are constantly required to gain ground in the endless struggle to preserve health and prolong life? Do at least some of the causes lie in the supposed waste and inefficiency of a highly fractionated health care delivery system? Are health care costs so high because people who do not have to pay their own health care bills out-of-pocket are overusing health care services? Are some providers reaping unconscionable profits? Is it a combination of these and other more possible causes that is driving up the cost of health care at an alarming rate?

Most people have opinions about the reasons for the rapid rise in health care costs, and some can argue their opinions convincingly and at great length. However, it is clearly evident that arguments alone and even arguments plus limited action have done little to stem the alarming rate of increase in health care costs.

FORCES FUELING HEALTH CARE COST INFLATION

The generally acknowledged causes of health care cost inflation, both real and perceived, include:

- increased hospital-day rates, stemming from increases in the costs of providing all hospital services and supporting the delivery of those services;
- increased use of laboratory tests, X-rays, drugs, pharmaceuticals and other ancillary services, and the increased cost of these basic services;
- increases in the number of procedures medically prescribed for each patient, including significant increases in the total number of surgeries performed;
- steady increases in physicians' charges;
- overexpansion of hospital facilities and duplication of hospital facilities and services;
- advancing medical technology, as more sophistication in equipment and skilled labor are brought to bear on health problems and more resources are applied to specific emerging medical needs of the population;
- increasingly larger and more numerous malpractice settlements, and corresponding increases in malpractice insurance premiums for provider organizations and individual medical practitioners;
- increasing costs of operating various government agencies, as more and more such agencies get deeper into the business of regulating health care quality and cost; and
- the alleged overuse of the health care system primarily by consumers but also by some providers, and the supposed abuse of some medical insurance programs.

It is popular practice for the various participants in the health care system—individual providers, provider organizations, payers, regulators and consumers—to blame each other for the largest part of the increase in health care costs. Although the system's participants can argue, perhaps forever, about who is at fault, the reality of the total increase in health care costs nevertheless remains to be reckoned with. Ultimately, it is the health care provider, whether individual or institutional, who is required to deal most directly with growing health care costs.

COST CONTAINMENT PRESSURES

There are a number of pressures, some independent of each other but most interrelated, that bear on the institutional provider of health care. Health care institutions are receiving a clear message—without also receiving any clear indication of means—to slow the rate of growth in the health care bill and to contain costs. These pressures on the health care institution are being applied by:

- employers, who pay a large share of increasing health care costs through health insurance premiums and the direct costs of company-sponsored health care plans;

- government, which pays a significant share of increasing health care costs with tax revenues;
- labor unions, many of which are seeing their members losing ground in the area of health benefits by having to directly bear a larger portion of increasing health care costs;
- consumer groups, collectives of citizens reacting to dramatic increases in the cost of an essential service; and
- taxpayer groups, collectives of citizens who see their taxes related to health care increasing without equivalent increases in the benefits received.

All of the foregoing pressures come to bear on the health care provider, the individual health care institution. The individual institution remains charged with the task of providing top-quality health care, including the provision of all new technology that could possibly have a positive impact on the restoration of health and the protection and extension of life, and of doing so while containing the increase in health care costs.

Although cost containment pressures are directed at the institution as a whole, within the health care institution these pressures must ultimately come to bear on those individuals who actively control or influence the expenditure of health care dollars. Specifically, cost containment

pressures are ultimately focused on the point at which ground-level action must be taken to control costs—the individual department manager or cost center supervisor.

EMPLOYER REACTION TO SPIRALING COSTS

From the mid-1960s or earlier until the early 1980s, many employers left the management of health care costs primarily to health insurance carriers. The majority of health insurance premiums were established by a standard markup over the long-run cost of claims. Insurance carriers profited from increasing health care costs, because a percentage markup applied to a larger base yielded a larger profit. Viewed in terms of how insurance carriers operated, there appeared to be an incentive to provide more and costlier service and thus a disincentive to adopt cost-saving practices.

Employers pay the largest share of the health care bill through health insurance premiums paid on behalf of employees. Health insurance costs were once a budget item of no particular significance to most business organizations. Because of dramatic increases in health care costs, this is no

Health insurance costs were once a budget item of no particular significance to most business organizations. Because of dramatic increases in health care costs, this is no longer the case.

longer the case. Health insurance premium costs are now significant items of cost to most companies.

During 1982 and 1983, health care cost inflation occurred at the rate of 15 to 20 percent.[7] In light of this double-digit inflation, employers began to feel the financial pinch associated with health care costs and began to shift more of these costs to their employees. As a result, during 1982 and 1983 increases in health insurance premium costs borne by employees averaged 20 to 40 percent.[8]

Overall, the efforts of employers to reduce the budgetary impact of escalating health care insurance premium costs have included:

- increasing the share of the premium costs for employees who pay for a portion of their own health insurance coverage through payroll deduction;
- establishing an employee share of the health insurance premium cost where none existed before;
- calling for employees to bear the full impact of future increases in health insurance premiums, thus requiring employees to pay an increasing proportion of premium costs as these costs grow;
- establishing absolute dollar caps on employer contributions; and
- requiring employees to pay larger health care plan deductibles.

All of the foregoing serve to pass on an ever-larger part of the increasing financial burden of health care to employees. Generally, employees are being required by employers to pay more and more for health care coverage.

Actions that may be seen by many companies as part of their necessary cost containment efforts are viewed by employees as direct losses of disposable income. Furthermore, in unionized companies such actions are seen by bargaining units as the intended results of take-away bargaining, having the effect of shifting the burden of health care premium costs from employer to employees.

If nothing else, the direct impact of employer reactions on spiraling health care costs has been a heightening of awareness of the health care cost issue. It could even be said that the intense interest of all concerned parties is arising because of a most effective stimulus to education on the part of both employers and employees—a direct impact on the pocketbook.

EMPLOYEE RESPONSE TO HEALTH CARE BENEFIT COST CUTTING

It is certainly not unusual for someone who once received something for free but who now must pay for it, or for someone who sees the accustomed cost of basic coverage or service increasing markedly, to react with complaints. Rapid health care cost increases and numerous employers' responses to such increases have caused many individual voices to be added to the general outcry concerning health care costs. In many instances, cost increases and employer responses have given rise to the vocal objections of labor unions.

Bargaining efforts

To a considerable extent, labor unions are in the forefront of organized opposition to the shifting of health insurance premium increases to employees. In December 1983 the Service Employees International Union (SEIU) announced the commencement of a national effort to counter rising health care costs and oppose what has been described as increasing management attacks on health care benefits. This particular union has gone on record as encouraging Blue Cross and Blue Shield to link premium rates to formal cost containment efforts, and it has also proposed to freeze physicians' fees.[9]

The SEIU has identified ten states as targets for its efforts: California, Georgia, Illinois, Missouri, Michigan, New York, Ohio, Oregon, Pennsylvania and Texas. The union's approach will be to encourage the passage of legislation aimed at freezing rates and fees until insurers can meet specific cost containment standards and until reasonable physician fee schedules can be negotiated with physicians. The union elected to focus efforts at the state legislative level because of their belief that the federal government has consistently refused to adopt national cost containment legislation.

SEIU has invited other unions to join in the effort to work toward retaining workers' health care coverage through tougher collective bargaining and through more direct involvement in the passage of regulatory legislation. In general, the unions have pointed out that:

- There are no clearly definite plans in the works to cap physicians' fees.
- There is essentially no limit on capital expansion and on equipment purchases by providers, except in a few states.
- There are inadequately few requirements for insurance carriers to adopt cost-saving practices.

The union position suggests that true health care cost containment will require:

- more efficient administration of insurance plans than is prevalent;
- discontinuance of unnecessary medical procedures;
- vastly increased utilization of alternatives to hospitalization; and
- adoption of flat fee schedules and competitive bidding for "hospitals, clinics, medical groups and individual doctors."[10]

Overall, most unions can be expected to engage in considerably tougher bargaining over health care benefits. Their objective will generally not be to acquire further gains, but rather to prevent further losses.

New options

Unions and other employee and consumer groups, plus selected arms of government and certain interested health care providers, are encouraging the health care system to turn toward:

- an increasing emphasis on preventive medicine;
- use of mandatory second opinions regarding the necessity of surgery;
- further shifting to the utilization of alternatives to hospitalization;
- means of further reducing the length of hospital stays;
- organized enhancement and support of self-help programs to assist people in dealing with hypertension, alcoholism, diabetes and other chronic ailments; and
- implementation of new programs intended to reduce and control occupational health and safety hazards.

Relative to a working individual's earnings, the health care coverage costs for many employees are no longer negligible. As these costs are a major and growing budget item for businesses, so are they a cost element precipitating increasing anxiety for individuals. Individuals are likely to continue to be concerned, especially as long as health care costs grow out of proportion to other costs of living.

FOCUS OF COST CONTAINMENT PRESSURE

In the view of some people, any organization or individual that renders bills for providing a health-related service is automatically responsible for at least part of the cost escalation problem. Most frequently tagged with such responsibility are the direct, hands-on providers of health care services, both organizations and individuals, and especially hospitals and physicians.

Hospitals and physicians

The hospital is frequently seen as a complex organization that is continually and arbitrarily charging more than necessary for a vital service that is needed by people who have few, if any, alternatives to using that service. The hospital is often seen as a rich organization; critics do not readily understand how this organization could absorb such large sums of money without having plenty left over. It is not unusual for a hospital's credibility regarding its true financial state to be quite low with many users of its services.

Physicians are viewed by many people as high-income earners who also seem to arbitrarily charge more than necessary for the provision of a vital service that is required by people who have few alternatives. In brief, the hospital and the physician are both frequently seen as charging more solely because their services are essential and there are no ready alternatives.

Certainly hospital and physician costs are necessarily the cost elements of the greatest concern in the health care system. In 1980 hospital charges accounted for 40.3 percent of all health care expenditures in the country, by far the largest share of the health care dollar. During the same year, physician charges accounted for

18.9 percent of the health care dollar. By comparison, the third largest component of cost in 1980 was nursing home care, consuming 8.4 percent of the health care dollar.[11]

Reimbursement regulations

It was once unthinkable to imagine that serious steps would ever be taken to cap health care expenditures, to actually place a limit on the amount of money flowing into the system. Capping, it was reasoned by many, would inevitably lead to cutbacks in service and to the overall erosion of the quality of health care. However, capping health care expenditures is precisely what is being done by way of various reimbursement regulations. Indeed, reimbursement regulations imposed on the health care system have one major ultimate net effect: They force changes to occur within the system by limiting the inflow of the system's primary resource, the money that is required to operate.

In a number of ways, external regulation has guaranteed chaos within the system. Consider thousands of hospitals and tens of thousands of other providers, all participating in a loosely defined "system" composed of countless cottage-industry elements, with this system supported in its entirety by seemingly runaway cost inflation. Pressure is then applied by capping the cost of the system and limiting the rate of cost growth by regulating the input of the system's critical resource—money.

The numerous elements making up the system respond to this pressure in a variety of ways:

- Some providers change in character as to the services they provide or the particular markets they serve. For example, a particular hospital, feeling the financial pinch, might abandon maternity services, a money-losing operation that is perhaps more efficiently provided by another institution, and turn attention to same-day surgery.
- Some providers, unable to adjust to the changing financial environment, may voluntarily or involuntarily go bankrupt and eventually leave the system.
- Some providers may merge or otherwise affiliate with other providers, reducing the total number of health care provider organizations but adding to the total number of institutions involved in multihospital systems.
- Some providers may take steps to achieve higher levels of internal operating efficiency so as to adjust to the decline in the financial resources available.

Drastic changes

Certainly, drastic changes have occurred in the United States health care system since external pressure began to be applied to hospitals. In 1968 there were 7,991 hospitals in the country; by 1979 the number of hospitals had dropped to 7,085, a decline of 11.3 percent in 11 years.[12]

Further change is expected in the number of active hospitals. It has been estimated, for instance, that the impact of the federal government's diagnosis related group reimbursement system may lead to the closure of one out of every five existing hospitals during the first five years of the system's implementation.[13]

Beyond a certain level of satisfaction of intellectual curiosity, there is no pressing need to pursue herein all of the possible ways in which the health care system may respond to current and emerging financial pressures. The shape and direction of most institutional responses will lie well beyond the control of the individual supervisor or manager within the institution. Rather, the primary interest in this discussion lies in how the individual supervisor's work is affected and in what the supervisor can do about mounting cost containment pressure.

HEALTH CARE COST CONTAINMENT: HERE TO STAY

The U.S. health care environment has changed dramatically in two critical, interrelated dimensions: the imposition of financial limitations on the system and the advent of open competition.

Simply stated, the amount of money devoted to health care is not being allowed to increase at a rate determined by the perceived needs of the system itself. The rate of growth is deliberately being slowed by the external imposition of regulatory

The U.S. health care environment has changed dramatically in two critical, interrelated dimensions: the imposition of financial limitations on the system and the advent of open competition.

mechanisms intended to stem the rise in the nation's health care bill by forcing changes to occur within the system.

Once almost universally discouraged and even today denied and regarded as harmful by some to the provision of quality health care, open competition among health care providers is on the increase. It is likely to attain considerable intensity for several years to come as the health care system shakes out and adjusts to external financial pressures.

In addition to regulatory pressure, there are other signs suggesting the growth of conditions favoring competition. For example, the United States is clearly headed into a period of oversupply of physicians. During the 1970s the number of physicians in the United States increased by 41 percent, a rate far outdistancing the growth of the general population.[14] There have been undeniable increases in the numbers of physicians relative to patients. The average available patients per physician dropped 21 percent from 1970 to 1983, and this ratio is expected to drop another 20 percent by 1990.[15]

Unused hospital capacity will become more significant as further options to short-term hospitalization are vigorously pursued for the sake of institutional survival. In spite of the previously noted decline in the number of hospitals, and occasional problems of geographic distribution of facilities, there remains considerable unused capacity within the hospital system. The health care providers that remain viable in the long run will be those who are able to provide quality care at competitive prices.

IMPLICATIONS FOR THE SUPERVISOR

The hospital is in a unique position, both as a health care provider with a strong interest in maintaining the level of income necessary to provide its service and remain solvent, and as an employer caught up in the necessity of paying an increasing health care bill for a number of employees. Certainly, the cost of employee health care coverage is fully as significant a budget item for a hospital as it is for a manufacturing or commercial enterprise with an equivalent number of employees. However, the manufacturing or commercial enterprise has only the interest, as far as health care is concerned, of stopping the growth in the amount paid for health care coverage.

The hospital would seem to be involved in a rather elementary conflict, on the one hand feeling the need to stem the growth of the bill for employee health care coverage, and on the other hand desiring to sustain the growth in income perceived as required to maintain operations. Addressing this basic conflict should ordinarily call for little involvement by the individual cost center supervisor.

The individual departmental or cost center supervisor is perhaps not involved in global matters of health care finance or in adjusting to competitive forces, marketing health care services and realigning the services of the organization. Nevertheless, that supervisor has an important role—perhaps the key role—in health care cost containment. The impact of the organization's goals on the actions of the individual supervisor at the department or cost center level must be considered.

Hospital costs are distributed among various components of expense approximately as follows:
- wages and salaries, 50 percent;
- employee benefits, 8 percent;
- contracted services, 7 percent;
- professional fees, 6 percent;
- capital expenditures, 6 percent;
- fuel and utilities, 6 percent;
- drugs and pharmaceuticals, 5 percent;
- food, 4 percent;
- medical supplies, 3 percent; and
- all other expenses, 5 percent.[16]

Although a few of these cost elements lie largely or perhaps completely beyond the individual supervisor's control, at the department or cost center level most of these costs can be controlled or at least influenced by the actions of the supervisor. Thus the institution's success at controlling costs will largely be the sum of the successful efforts of individual supervisors. Certainly, the most effective control is that exercised at the point in the organization where the resources are actually applied.

The pass-through concept of pricing health care services—that is, the "cost–plus" approach—calls for all actual costs of providing service, plus a markup for profit, surplus or to cover bad debts or whatever else may not be covered, to be passed directly through to the ultimate payer, who then pays without question. This is largely a practice of the past. It has always been the function of the health care supervisor to assure the delivery of quality patient care. It is now the function of the health care supervisor, and is likely to be for the foreseeable future, to assure the delivery of this quality care in a cost-effective manner.

It has long been the attitude of many in health care that control of costs automatically leads to diminution of quality, that it is not possible to focus seriously on cost control and productivity improvement without impairing the organization's ability to sustain high quality. However, this attitude appears based on two implicit, and generally fallacious, assumptions.

The first is that there is a direct relationship between quality and cost. (Lowest quality equates to lowest cost, higher quality means higher cost and highest quality means highest cost.) The second is that the present way of doing things represents the highest quality available for the money. (This is the belief that it is not possible to improve today's cost picture without adversely affecting quality, and that it is not possible to increase quality without increasing cost.)

Regardless of an individual's position relative to the quality–versus–cost issue, some undeniable forces have entered the health care system:

- Health care costs are being capped and will not be allowed to grow unchecked.
- Competition will become a way of life in health care.
- Continued high–quality care will be demanded in spite of pressures to contain costs.

As they have long been in many industries other than health care, the control of costs and the enhancement of productivity will henceforth be critical elements of every supervisor's job.

REFERENCES

1. U.S. Bureau of the Census. *Health Care Expenditures.* Washington, D.C.: GPO, 1980.
2. Ibid.
3. Ibid.

4. Gibson, R.M., and Waldo, D.R. "National Health Expenditures," *Health Care Financing Review.* Office of Research, Demonstrations, and Statistics, Health Care Financing Adminis-

tration, HCFA Pub. No. 03123. Washington, D.C.: Government Printing Office, September 1981.

5. Bureau of National Affairs. "Business, Labor Search for Solutions to Spiraling Health Care Expense." *White Collar Report* 54 (December 14, 1983): 558.

6. American Society for Personnel Administration. *Resource* (February 1984): 2.

7. Schoen, C. "Maintaining and Improving Health Benefits by Containing Costs." *White Collar Report*, Bureau of National Affairs. 54 (December 7, 1983): 535.

8. Ibid.

9. Bureau of National Affairs. "SEIU Plan to Press for Legislation on Cost Containment." *White Collar Report* 54 (December 7, 1983): 518–19.

10. Ibid., 518–19.

11. Gibson and Waldo, "National Health Expenditures."

12. U.S. National Center for Health Statistics. As cited in *1983 Health Care Executive's Appointment Book*. Rockville, Md.: Aspen Systems, 1983.

13. Beck, D.F. "The Hospital's Financial Future: DRGs and Beyond." *The Health Care Supervisor* 3 (January 1985): 1–11.

14. U.S. National Center for Health Statistics.

15. Schoen, "Maintaining and Improving Health Benefits by Containing Costs," 536.

16. Johnson, K.A., and Neely, C. "Hospital Economic Forecast." *Hospitals* 57 (October 1, 1983): 87.

Survival through productivity improvement

Donald F. Beck
President
D.F. Beck & Associates
Memphis, Tennessee

Jack Dempsey
Assistant Professor
University of Tennessee Center for
  Health Sciences
Memphis, Tennessee

AMERICAN HOSPITALS are under increasing pressure to become more productive. The pressure is especially strong in the rural hospitals and in the high percentage Medicare and Medicaid hospitals. The current reimbursement environment has been especially unfavorable to these hospitals.

Hospitals have entered bankruptcy and yet had excess staff; hospitals have closed when all they needed to do to survive was to appropriately reduce staff size. We all know of hospitals that were losing hundreds of thousands of dollars, were taken over by new owners or new managers, and within a year had realized net incomes of hundreds of thousands of dollars. This seems like a dichotomy but, when we examine the facts more closely, it makes good sense. Before prospective payment the economic incentives for hospitals were similar to those of government agencies. As a result, many departments became as unproductive as comparative departments in government agencies.

Health Care Superv, 1991, 10(1), 1–13
©1991 Aspen Publishers, Inc.

Personnel in overstaffed departments work long, hard hours. Often they require significant overtime just to keep up with the workload. They do not waste time. They waste effort on marginally useful tasks—sometimes counter-productive tasks—or by pushing work through an ineffective work flow system. After years of ineffective work flow, people naturally lose their perspective on what constitutes normal. They truly believe that what they are experiencing is the norm, except that they are understaffed.

Occasionally in government a legislature or other authority will take a detached perspective and drastically cut a budget or eliminate a department. The same happens in hospitals. A new owner, a new administrator, or an incumbent administrator will take a detached perspective and drastically reduce staff size. Often a consultant is used to remove bias and assure that there is a detached perspective.

The budget process normally takes the status quo and makes adjustments. An industrial engineer does the same through a more orderly process. Industrial engineering processes, however, normally use historical work flow, historical staffing, and historical tasks as a starting point. They are biased and do not take a detached perspective. This article, which presents two case studies and numerous examples, will show a department director who is willing to take a detached perspective how to recognize moderate and severe overstaffing.

HOW OVERSTAFFING EVOLVES

Employees have an innate need to be busy and productive. If there are too many employees, they will adjust the system until everyone is busy. Often the supervisor will see that the workload is falling behind and another employee is added, then the system adjusts again so that everyone is busy. Work expands to consume the time and personnel available. If the economic incentives support this scenario over a period of many years, this staffing pattern becomes the norm for that institution notwithstanding the norm for the identical function at other hospitals. This point will become clear from the case studies presented later in this article.

As the American economy has moved from a manufacturing economy to a service-based economy, management has struggled to adapt production methods to service industries. Contrary to financial principles, we have substituted labor for capital in the labor-intensive health care industry. The result is a health care system that absorbed up to 13 percent of the gross national product (GNP) in 1990. Evolving health care technology has resulted in a less efficient and less effective system because of the failure to develop quality control standards. Each new device or test adds to an already inefficient system. Physicians are often uncertain whether they are doing the right thing because clinical standards are difficult to establish in this turbulent health care environment.

A solution lies in the development of a standard cost accounting system based on currently attainable standards to improve productivity. This system may be derived from historical data, time-and-motion studies, or engineering estimates. Historical data are the least desirable but the easiest to obtain. A standard cost accounting system based on industry health care norms may be the most desirable. These data, however, are often not available because hospitals will not share cost data for competitive reasons or because there are no data due to inadequate accounting systems. Also, rapidly changing technology means rapidly changing costs.

In one example, an executive came to a

hospital system from another industry. He initiated a new financial analysis department. This department had five staff members, each with a master's degree in business administration, and several support staff. Within two months this department, whose function did not previously exist, was working weekends to keep up. It was producing a budget variance report for each hospital in the system that consisted of more than 100 typed pages, delineating budget variances for each department. To those not directly involved this is obviously a counterproductive task: it requires considerable effort on the part of department directors in addition to the effort of the financial analysis staff, and it is such a meticulous delineation of budget variances it would never be read by top executives. To those directly involved, however, this department's activities were not seen as counterproductive. The inappropriate staffing and activity levels became the norm for this system.

One hospital was a debtor in possession under the protection of federal bankruptcy court. The hospital was still losing money and believed that changes in the reimbursement system were responsible. Because of a detached perspective, consultants were able to reduce staff size by a third. The local paper carried articles describing how disastrous the new staffing was. There was some resistance from the medical staff, and several department directors quit. There was no problem replacing the department directors who left, medical staff members became complacent, and the local newspaper went on to cover other issues. Within six months, the hospital was profitable.

At another hospital the new owners immediately cut two people from every department. This was a one-time measure, after which other cuts were made. At the time of the takeover, some departments only had one or two em-

ployees; accordingly, these departments were eliminated. As a direct result of the decision to arbitrarily cut two full-time equivalents (FTEs) from every department, three department directors resigned; the hospital replaced these directors without incident. Six months later, operations were normal even though additional cutbacks had been made and the departments that had been eliminated at the change of ownership were not reinstated.

This is not to advocate arbitrary cuts in staff size, nor to advocate even significant cuts in staff size. These examples are provided to show that personnel adjust to reductions as well as to increases in staffing in a surprisingly short period of time. The systems, work flow, and number of tasks adjust until everyone is busy. There is a point in staffing where additional personnel become wasteful and another point where they become counterproductive. It is the responsibility of management to recognize the staffing level that optimizes both patient care and net income.

It is the responsibility of management to recognize the staffing level that optimizes both patient care and net income.

The following paragraphs present a case study, followed by tools that can be used to find optimal staffing point. This discussion will be followed by a more detailed case study and more tools to use to find optimal staffing levels. All of the case studies, as well as the examples used in this article, are true. Nothing has been fabricated. The case studies represent actual data from calendar year 1988.

CASE STUDY: SMALL HOSPITAL

A 95-bed hospital has the following statistics for the year: acute care days, 12,096; intensive care unit (ICU) days, 1,119; total care days (acute plus ICU), 13,215; and admissions, 1,463. The administrator holds a master's degree in public health and one in health services administration. He has been the administrator of this hospital since 1983. Prior experience includes the position of assistant administrator at two different California hospitals and associate administrator at a complex that included a chemical dependency unit. The controller has a degree in accounting. He has been a hospital controller since 1982. He has worked at three hospitals, but most of his experience has been gained at the current facility.

The on-site administrative staff has been under great financial pressure. Staff members believe, and have stated emphatically, that expenses have been cut as much as possible. They have spent many long days on budgets. Table 1 presents current staffing. It represents a significant decrease in FTEs from the previous year.

It would be best for the reader to take some time to analyze this hospital before reading the following analysis. There is not a great deal of information for this facility, so the analysis should be simple.

The first point to note is that the average daily census is 36. This hospital is in an overbedded area, and the probability of the census growing is remote. Therefore, this hospital should be viewed as a 45-bed facility with an average occupancy of 85 percent. There are certain attributes of a 95-bed hospital that 45-bed hospitals do not have. As long as management views itself as running a 95-bed facility rather than one of 45, it will not find all of the excess staffing.

There are 9 FTEs in nursing administration, and with the inservice educator there are 10 FTEs. The national average for nursing administration is 6 percent of total nursing staff. Using 6 percent there would be 4.5 FTEs in nursing administration rather than 10. However, 45-bed facilities normally have less than 4 FTEs in nursing administration. For facilities this size 2 FTEs are common. It can be assumed that this hospital has from 5.5 to 8.0 FTEs excess in nursing administration.

The ICU uses almost 32 hours of paid time per patient per day. This is 1.25 FTEs per patient, 24 hours per day. At a hospital of this size, patients, even those in ICU, are not sick enough to need this much care.

Surgery and recovery uses 17.8 paid hours per admission. Assuming half the admissions receive surgery (a reasonable assumption), then there are almost 36 paid hours per surgery. From a detached perspective, it is obvious that surgery is grossly overstaffed. Those closer to the situation cannot see this because the personnel are probably busy most of the time.

Respiratory therapy consumes 1.3 paid hours per patient day, and ECG uses almost 40 minutes per day. Dietary and cafeteria uses 40 minutes of paid time per patient meal. Because of the all-important detached perspective, the consultants (or other outsiders) can see this overstaffing.

Administration has 5 FTEs, including two assistant administrators and two clerical personnel. Most 45-bed hospitals do not have even one assistant administrator; two is gross waste. Admitting uses almost three paid hours per admission, while purchasing has three full-time people for a 45-bed hospital. The business office consumes almost 13 paid hours per discharge in a highly computerized hospital.

Finally, housekeeping and maintenance often have approximately the same number of

Table 1. Current staffing

Department	FTEs	Statistics
Nursing administration	9.0	7–10 FTEs
Inservice education	1.0	
Medical-surgical nursing	34.0	5.8 hr/day
ICU	17.0	31.6 hr/day
Surgery and recovery	12.5	17.8 hr/admission
Emergency	7.0	17.8 hr/admission
Central supply	3.0	0.5 hr/day
Laboratory	12.0	1.9 hr/day
Radiology	9.0	1.4 hr/day
Pharmacy	3.0	0.5 hr/day
Respiratory therapy	8.0	1.3 hr/day
ECG	4.0	0.6 hr/day
Physical therapy	2.0	2.8 hr/admission
Medical record	5.5	7.8 hr/admission
Social services	1.0	1.4 hr/admission
Administration	5.0	7.1 hr/admission
Business office	9.0	12.8 hr/admission
Accounting	3.0	4.3 hr/admission
Admitting	2.0	2.8 hr/admission
Purchasing	3.0	0.5 hr/day
Data processing	3.0	4.3 hr/day
Communications	2.5	0.4 hr/day
Dietary and cafeteria	10.0	0.7 hr/meal
Housekeeping	6.5	1.0 hr/day
Plant operations/maintenance	13.0	2.0 hr/day
Total	185.0	

employees. When this is not the case, one has to look closely to determine why. This hospital has 6.5 personnel in housekeeping and 13 in maintenance. It appears that maintenance is overstaffed. This total may, perhaps, include security or parking garage cashiers. However, since maintenance has twice as many personnel as housekeeping, it should be studied closely.

In a very short period of time this analysis has identified some conservative cuts that can be made. They are summarized in Table 2.

After studying the departments more closely, it may become clear that all of the reductions delineated above cannot be made. However, this first draft of cuts is conservative and all of the departments have not been studied. This hospital is struggling to survive, and it blames

Table 2. Potential reductions by position or department

	No. of Department	Annual salary with fringe benefits reductions ($)	Total cost ($)
Nursing administration	6	30,000	180,000
ICU	5	28,000	140,000
Surgery and recovery	6	28,000	168,000
Respiratory and ECG	6	23,000	138,000
Dietary	3	18,000	54,000
Medical record	3	20,000	60,000
Administration	2	35,000	70,000
Business office	5	18,000	90,000
Admitting	1	18,000	18,000
Purchasing	1	18,000	18,000
Switchboard	2	18,000	36,000
Maintenance	6	20,000	120,000
Total			$1,092,000

prospective payment, physicians, and third party payors. However, the real reason it is suffering is that it is paying out more than $1 million per year in wages plus benefits to personnel who are not productive.

BEGIN TO IDENTIFY STAFFING

There are three simple points in identifying overstaffing. In order of importance, they are
1. reduce all financial information to a ratio,
2. spread the comparison over time, and
3. compare the ratio to an outside indicator.

Reducing information to a ratio is by far the most important task. This is not just true of personnel costs. It is true of balance sheets, income statements, and virtually all financial information. We cannot understand only dollars; money must be compared to something to

become meaningful. Consider the budget information for an outpatient clinic presented in Table 3.

Table 3 may be called a "Gee Whiz Report." The reader does not know what it means to have a $10,000 personnel expense variance because of not understanding dollars. Pure dollars alone have no meaning. The reader also does not know what a revenue variance or supply variance means. All one can say is "Gee whiz, I didn't know that" or "Gee whiz, that's interesting." By itself, the information in this type of report is not meaningful. Normally readers start to think about information in com-

We cannot understand only dollars; money must be compared to something to become meaningful.

Table 3. Outpatient clinic budget information

	Current month			Year to date		
Account	Actual ($)	Budgeted ($)	Variance ($)	Actual ($)	Budgeted ($)	Variance ($)
Revenue	4,100	4,500	(400)	19,500	18,000	1,500
Expenses						
Personnel	2,487	2,500	(13)	12,876	10,000	2,876
Supplies	876	1,000	(124)	4,600	4,000	600
Other	384	500	(116)	1,632	2,000	(368)
Total expenses	3,747	4,000	(253)	19,108	16,000	3,108
Net gain (loss)	353	500	(147)	392	2,000	(1,608)

parative or ratio terms. Once thoughts become ratio oriented, dollars start to become meaningful (see Table 4).

The first line is a statistic; all other lines relate to this statistic. A one dollar variance in salary expense per clinic visit—whether this is a positive or negative variance—is meaningful. One knows what it means to have a two dollar per clinic visit variance in revenue, however, a $10,000 revenue variance is just a gee whiz statement.

Every hospital department should monitor the following ratios on a regular basis:
- productive hours to paid hours,
- average hourly pay rate, and
- paid hours per defined work unit.

The defined work unit is whatever is available and appropriate for that department. Some examples of work units are shown in the Box. For any department in which a work unit is not readily available, use adjusted patient days (APD). APD, which is the default statistic for

Table 4. Outpatient clinic information in comparative or ratio terms

	Current month			Year to date		
Description	Actual	Budgeted	Variance	Actual	Budgeted	Variance
Clinic visits	97	90	7	418	360	58
Per clinic visit ($)						
Revenue	42	50	(8)	47	50	(3)
Salary	26	28	(2)	31	28	3
Supply	9	11	(2)	11	11	
Other	4	6	(2)	4	6	(2)
Net gain (loss) ($)	3	5	(2)	1	5	(4)

Examples of Work Units

Department	Unit
Laboratory	CAPs
Radiology	Relative value unit
Physical therapy	Modualities
Maintenance	Building gross square feet
Housekeeping	Square feet serviced
Surgery	Hours

---

all hospital departments, is calculated as follows:

$$APD = \frac{\text{Total patient revenue}}{\text{Inpatient revenue}} \times \text{Patient days}$$

The formula adjusts patient days for outpatient activity. If 10 percent of the revenue is outpatient activity, then the formula grosses up patient days by 10 percent.

CASE STUDY: MEDIUM SIZE HOSPITAL

This hospital believes that the third party payor system is responsible for its poor financial plight. However, using the detached perspective, the real culprit is overstaffing.

This facility is licensed for 680 beds but is operating only 400 beds at this time. It considers itself a 400-bed hospital. It is an old hospital in an economically depressed area of a large city; it is about 60 percent Medicare and Medicaid. Of the 40 percent balance, half are written off as uncollectible. The hospital receives full billed charges for only 20 percent of its patient revenue.

The facility has installed an elaborate acuity profile system to help in nurse staffing, has a very detailed and intense budget process, has provided a long list of what it considers

cost-cutting initiatives recently initiated, and has made all of the apparent right moves. Management honestly believes it has cut staff as lean as possible.

Some statistics for this hospital for the past year are as follows: acute care days, 94,006; intensive care days, 10,169; nursery days, 0; total days (acute plus intensive care plus nursery), 104,175; and admissions, 6,449. The nursery was closed in a prior year as a cost-cutting measure. Staffing statistics per paid hour are provided in Table 5.

This hospital is in serious financial trouble; it may not survive. Taking a detached perspective, several examples of gross overstaffing are readily seen. The first obvious overstaffed department is the clinic, using 2.7 paid hours per visit. Clinic visits are scheduled and therefore do not involve waiting time to the extent of the emergency department. A physician with one assistant could only see three patients per day with a productivity rate of 2.7 paid hours per visit.

Surgery uses 8.2 paid hours per surgery hour; the recovery room uses 3.4 paid hours per recovery room hour. Both are clear examples of overstaffing when reduced to ratios.

The laboratory consumes 3.2 paid hours per patient day. (It is better to use College of American Pathologists (CAP) units if they are available.) The national average for a laboratory is 1.3 paid hours per patient day. ECG uses 0.3 paid hours per patient day, which is almost enough time for every patient to receive an ECG every day.

The cardiac catheterization laboratory consumes more than 14 paid hours per procedure. The low number of procedures suggests that the system is so inefficient that physicians are sending patients elsewhere for this procedure. This is an example of overstaffing that has become counterproductive.

It is especially interesting to observe the administration and fiscal departments. It is

Table 5. Staffing statistics per paid hour

Department	FTEs	Workload measure	Statistics/ hour
Routine nursing	326	94,006 patient days	7.2
Intensive care	90	10,169 patient days	18.4
Emergency	24	19,305 visits	2.6
Clinic	20	15,475 visits	2.7
Surgery	52	13,215 hours	8.2
Recovery	20	12,206 hours	3.4
Laboratory	146	94,006 patient days	3.2
ECG	14	94,006 patient days	0.3
Cardiac catheterization laboratory	9	1,320 procedures	14.2
Radiology	66	94,006 patient days	1.5
Computed tomography scanning	6	6,348 scans	2.0
Respiratory	38	94,006 patient days	0.8
Physical therapy	18	81,355 modualities	0.46
Dialysis	3	1,080 treatments	5.8
Other ancillary	6	94,006 patient days	0.13
Dietary	59	53,816 estimated meals	0.5
Cafeteria	28	1,398 employees	41.7
Laundry	5	94,006 patient days	0.11
Social work	8	6,499 discharges	2.6
Plant maintenance	43	90,542 square feet	82.1
Security and parking	32	90,542 square feet	61.1
Housekeeping	56	90,542 square feet	106.9
Central supply	16	54,980 costed requisitions	0.6
Pharmacy	28	363,040 costed requisitions	0.16
General accounting	16	400 beds	83.2
Patient accounting	61	6,499 discharges	19.5
Hospital administration	86	400 beds	447.2
Data processing	36	6,499 discharges	11.5
Purchasing/stores	13	94,006 patient days	0.3
Medical record	25	6,499 discharges	8.0
Medical staff	7	205 physicians	71.0
Medical review	9	205 physicians	91.3
Nursing administration	32	531 FTEs	125.3
Total	1,398		

difficult to imagine what 16 people in general accounting are spending their time on until one looks at the 36 people in data processing. A data processing staff of this size guarantees that the hospital's systems are complicated and cumbersome. Patient accounting uses almost 20 paid hours per discharge, which exceeds the amount of time it would take to process all billings by hand.

Hospital administration, with 86 FTEs, sets the tone for the rest of the hospital. When compared to other hospitals of this size, hospital administration is almost 70 FTEs too high. To the administration at this hospital there does not appear to be overstaffing because everyone is working hard. Most of the readers of this article will recognize that there have to be complicated processes, excess reporting, and many meetings at this hospital. This hospital probably cannot be successful until the administrator retires or is removed. At that time they would need to hire an outsider to correct the gross overstaffing.

It is relatively easy to identify more than $5 million in obvious staffing reductions that can be made. This hospital may close without recognizing how readily available financial success can be.

The following are some broad indicators to look for when studying a hospital. These indicators do not always hold true, but they are a starting point in hospitals being studied for the first time.

- If there are several laboratory departments overstaffing is common. Several laboratory departments would be, for example, chemistry, cytology, pathology, etc.
- If there are several radiology departments overstaffing is common. Several radiology departments would be, for example, nuclear medicine, ultrasound, computed tomography, diagnostic, etc.
- The fiscal area normally has some overstaffing in a hospital that has a full time financial officer. If the fiscal area includes very specialized departments that are not commonly found in other hospitals, these departments can most often be eliminated. Some examples of these are inter-

nal audit, reimbursement, and budget analysis.

- Maintenance and housekeeping often have the same number of FTEs. If one of these is significantly higher, then both should be studied closely.
- For hospitals of less than 50 beds, the decision to have a cafeteria should be studied carefully. Between 50 and 100 beds a cafeteria is often an unneeded expense. For larger hospitals a cafeteria is usually cost beneficial because it keeps employees on the premises during lunch and supper times.

MEASURING REPORTS

In productivity measuring, the most important point is to use ratios. Another important point is to compare these ratios over time. In the case studies it was shown how productivity ratios can identify severe overstaffing. To identify moderate overstaffing, the current productivity ratios are compared over time. Normally, when department productivity ratios are first employed, the department statistics for at least the past two years are calculated. Some examples of staffing reports over time are shown in Tables 6 and 7.

In productivity measuring, the most important point is to use ratios. Another important point is to compare these ratios over time.

Table 6 compares the seven acute care nursing units of a 238-bed hospital. There are many reasons why one nursing specialty floor could require more nursing time than another, but this is still an excellent comparison. It provides a starting point. Another comparative ratio re-

Table 6. Patient days by unit

Nursing unit	Beds	Patient days	Hours	Hours/day
1	22	6,200	46,872	7.56
2	36	11,100	75,702	6.82
3	36	11,700	67,509	5.77
4	36	11,000	112,530	10.23
5	36	12,600	98,406	7.81
6	36	10,400	100,360	9.65
7	36	11,000	90,420	8.22
Total	238	74,000	591,799	
Average				8.00

port is possible when the budget is established using productivity goals. In this scenario, it is possible to calculate an attainment index. Table 7 compares the attainment index for different hospital departments. This index can be shown for the current month, for the year to date, or both. Once it is put into a computer program different comparisons are relatively easy to make.

The second most effective tool in productivity measuring is to compare the ratio over time.

Table 8 shows the change in the measurement statistic as well as the change in the ratio.

Figure 1 depicts a staffing report that is relatively easy to calculate and provides additional information. The staffing for these three dissimilar types of care will be different. However, the change over time should be similar. If one grows at a rate significantly different, this should be investigated.

Comparative productivity ratios over time are an excellent way to determine whether one

Table 7. Attainment index by department

Department (ratio)	Goal	Actual	Attainment
Dietary (meals/hour)	3.0	2.8	0.93
Plant (hours/1,000 square feet)	20.0	21.5	1.08
Housekeeping (hours/100 square feet)	50.0	52.3	1.05
Operating room (hours/visit)	10.0	11.0	1.10
Laboratory (tests/hour)	5.0	5.5	1.10
Radiology (hours/procedure)	1.0	0.9	0.90
Obstetrics (hours/obstetrics patient day)	5.0	5.1	1.02
Medical-surgical nursing (hours/patient day)	5.0	4.8	0.96

Table 8. Comparative annual statistics

Period	Total patient days	Total nursing hours	Total nursing hours per patient day
1985	87,853	493,733.9	5.62
1986	84,185	536,258.5	6.37
1987	86,611	589,820.9	6.81
1988	88,493	635,379.7	7.18
1989	89,590	675,508.6	7.54

department in a comparative group is losing control. Some common comparisons include

- Different radiology departments such as radiology, ultrasound, and nuclear medicine;
- Different laboratory departments such as cystology, chemistry, and blood bank; and
- Different departments that use a common measurement statistic such as maintenance, housekeeping, and security.

The third and final test to measure productivity is to compare ratios to an outside source. By noting movement in a ratio over time one can tell how a department is adjusting to acuity or other factors. By noting the same ratio movement over time for an outside source, one can tell if the hospital has adjusted appropriately when compared to its peers in the same environment. The following example (see Figure 2) provides both an external comparison and a trend analysis. It shows how a department compares to a regional and a national average. In addition, it shows how changes in the productivity compared to those for regional and national counterparts. This analysis is extremely

Comparative Department Ratios
(paid hours per patient day)

Period	Medical-surgical	Obstetrics	Intensive care
1985			
1986			
1987			
1988			
1989			
1990			
Percent change			

Figure 1. Illustrative staffing report.

External Trend Analysis

Period	Nursing hours/ patient day	Regional index same bed size	National index same bed size
1985			
1986			
1987			
1988			
1989			
1990			
Percent change			

Figure 2. Illustrative report showing comparison to outside sources.

powerful and can be prepared for any department in which comparative statistics are available.

• • •

There are dozens of additional case studies as well as success stories. The number of ways in which the information can be presented is limited only by the creativity of the user.

In order of importance, the three principles remain

1. Convert all data to ratios.
2. Study emerging trends in the way the ratio changes over time.
3. Compare changes over time as well as static ratios to an outside source.

To begin this program one needs to see what information is available at a particular hospital. If no other acceptable statistic is available use adjusted patient days. It is important that a productivity tracking system not be delayed until a system for statistical reporting is developed. It is also important to keep the system simple.

Productivity monitoring is difficult because it requires a new perspective. We are used to using historical data and unique characteristics of a hospital in the budget process. Productivity gains require a detached perspective. Often only an outsider can identify some examples of overstaffing. The process is difficult, but it is not complicated.

Productivity experts tell us we can produce a service faster, cheaper, or better, but not all three. Health care quality control ensures a better service. A standard cost accounting system for the health care industry may provide a less expensive service through better cost control. Productivity—the ratio of work output to resource input (health care costs)—can be increased.

To make productivity improvement work the users must take the view of the entire institution rather than that of a department. Productivity measuring is necessary to ensure the survival of hospitals. This process could have saved many of the hospitals that were forced to close, and it could improve the financial health of many hospitals today.

Part II
Tackling Productivity Improvement

Human work performance: It's not as simple as you think

Richard G. Melecki
Manager
Organizational Effectiveness
    and Development
Kaiser Permanente
Cleveland, Ohio

"THEY ARE A TOUGH group," declared the director of medical records to the consultant.

"As I explained earlier, the purpose of this group is to code completed records for input into the computer. The hospital is then reimbursed by various third party payers on the basis of this information. It used to be that we could live with a backlog of 50 or so charts. However, this represents about $1 million in billing for the hospital. The vice president for finance recently told me to get the backlog down—or else."

"Do you have a work–output standard for these coders, and have they been meeting it?" asked the consultant.

"Our standard, which I developed based on my experience, is three records per hour. Nobody in the group has met this standard yet, although one person has come close a couple of times."

Health Care Superv, 1989, 7(2), 23–31
© 1989 Aspen Publishers, Inc.

After making a notation, the consultant asked, "What have you tried so far to reduce the backlog?"

"Well," responded the director, "at the request of the coders themselves, we improved their educational program. I have also tightened up on supervision, checking them more closely every day. So far, nothing seems to work in getting the backlog down."

"What I need from you," he continued to the consultant, "is a time study of the individual work–output standard. I am ready to start disciplinary action, and I want to make sure I win if we go to grievance. I am convinced it is time to fire some of these people and get coders in here who want to do the job."

• • •

Such dialogue is becoming all too familiar in the modern health care environment. Previous levels of work performance, acceptable in a time of cost–plus reimbursement, are no longer economically feasible for health care institutions.

Well-meaning managers often attempt to apply uncoordinated, single-focus solutions, such as education or motivational techniques, to complex work–performance problems. When this one-shot approach fails, as it often does, the manager is likely to become frustrated and move directly to disciplinary action.

The problem is that in complex organizations such as health care institutions, work-performance problems are also complex. Employees do not work in a vacuum. Rather, they depend on others for things

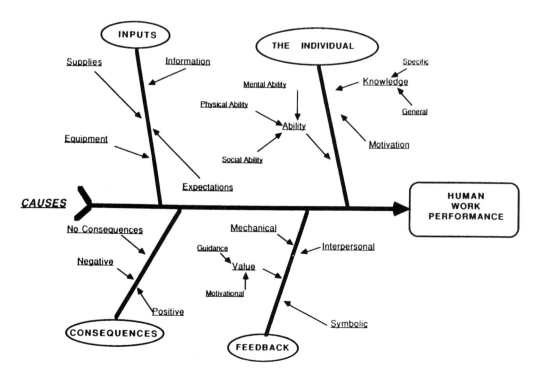

Figure 1. Human work performance: Cause and effect diagram.

such as information, raw materials, and feedback.

To ascribe an employee's poor work performance to a lack of motivation is often simplistic. The individual may, in fact, be highly motivated to do the job well. However, there may be other factors in the work environment that make it literally impossible to meet the supervisor's demands.

Firing poor performers before every possible barrier to effectiveness has been removed is both unfair and inhumane.

If individual work performance is not a simple phenomenon, what are the various factors that affect an employee's effectiveness on the job? One way to visualize this complex web of relationships is through a cause and effect (or "fishbone") diagram (Figure 1). Originally developed for use by Japanese quality circles, the diagram shows the factors that contribute to excellent work performance.[1]

Each "rib" of the fishbone diagram identifies a key variable that influences human work performance.

- Work inputs.
- Consequences (reward and punishments).
- The individual who does the job.
- Feedback.

These dominant variables are circled for emphasis. Each key variable has a variety of subfactors, which are connected to the appropriate rib of the fishbone by arrows. Some of these have, in turn, their own subfactors, also connected by arrows.

The objective—excellent human work performance—is listed at the box on the right-hand side. The stronger each factor is in a given work situation, the better the probability of high levels of performance.

Conversely, if the diagram is used as a starting point for analysis, it is possible to identify some of the potential causes of substandard performance.

WORK INPUTS

No one would expect a carpenter to build a house without nails or lumber, nor would this carpenter be likely to meet the builder's specifications without access to plans for the house. As Figure 2 suggests, both materials and information are key inputs into the carpenter's job performance.

The physical inputs to work performance are perhaps the most obvious. An employee must have the physical supplies and raw materials needed to do the job. The worker must also have the proper tools.

When the tools are simple, design is rarely an issue. After all, a hammer is not a very complex instrument. However, extremely sophisticated tools such as computers are more common in today's workplace. In recent years, much research has been done on the human-factors approach to designing complex equipment.[2]

Often less apparent as a key input into work performance is information. Gener-

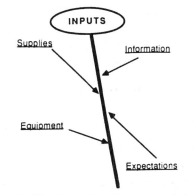

Figure 2. Key inputs into the carpenter's job include materials and information.

ally, information inputs fall into two categories: information about *what to do*—also called job expectations—and information about *how* to do the job. This latter type of information is used to guide performance.

There are a variety of strategies to correct a situation in which inadequate or ineffective inputs result in substandard employee performance. If the employee lacks basic materials, supplies, or information, it may be necessary to change work or information flows using some form of systems analysis to establish proper procedures.

Training, which is a knowledge-based strategy, can also be effective. It can show the employee how the job should be done and can help to establish management's expectations for performance.

CONSEQUENCES

Experimental evidence has repeatedly shown that people do things (or refrain from doing things) because certain consequences are likely to follow from their actions.

Experimental evidence has repeatedly shown that people do things (or refrain from doing things) because certain consequences are likely to follow from their actions.

Figure 3 suggests that when an employee behaves in a particular way on the job, there are three possible results from his or her point of view:

1. Something may happen that the employee likes (a positive consequence).
2. Something may happen that the em-

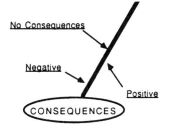

Figure 3. The employee believes that his or her behavior can result in one of three possible outcomes—positive consequence, negative consequence, or no consequence.

ployee does not like (a negative consequence).
3. Nothing at all may happen.

When something pleasant happens and the employee connects that experience with something he or she just did, there is a good chance that the employee will repeat the behavior again. On the other hand, if something happens that the employee does not like, or if nothing at all happens, there is a good chance that he or she will not repeat the action.

The wise supervisor, upon seeing the employee doing a job well tries to make something happen that the employee likes—for example, sincere praise the supervisor may give. At best, punishing employees through reprimands may stop what they are doing wrong—temporarily. Not paying attention to the good things an employee does decreases the chances that he or she will continue to perform well. Like snuffing out a candle, ignoring good performance extinguishes desirable job behavior.

Even more interestingly, some research suggests that the *expectation* of reward is itself motivating.[3] Most employees will work hard even though they only get paid every two weeks. It is not necessary to see each dollar as it is earned. Knowing that the paycheck will come when expected is itself a motivating factor.

This phenomenon points out the importance of consistency in supervisory behavior. The effective supervisor does not reward effective performance only some of the time, such as during an annual appraisal interview. He or she must be consistently rewarding, by regularly noting and praising desirable work performance, until the expectation of recognition for a job well done becomes itself rewarding to the employee.

This requires a level of self-discipline. Most supervisors are trained to look for the things that go wrong on the job. Very often this "management by exception" mentality leads them to note only the negatives in employee performance. It often requires a good deal of concentration to find the things that people do well on the job and then sincerely and deliberately to reward effective performance. However, when a supervisor does so, the results are almost magical. Sincere praise, such as verbal recognition, can be an extremely powerful motivator, especially when it is backed up by tangible rewards (e.g., pay raises).

Many performance problems result from inappropriate application of consequences by supervisors. Typically a supervisor may overuse punishment under the mistaken notion that "being tough" on employees gets the best job results. Or a supervisor may inadvertently punish good performance, as when the employee who finishes work early gets more to do as a "reward" for being efficient.

Unfortunately, instances of ineffective performance arise almost inevitably when supervisors ignore desirable job behaviors. When supervisors consciously or uncon-sciously follow the philosophy that "the squeaky wheel gets the oil," they may find that employees with problem behaviors get "oiled" by their attention most of the time. Productive employees—those who show up for work on time, pull their share of the load, and even help others in a pinch—are often ignored. An employee's good performance may diminish over a long period of time unless it is recognized and rewarded.

Whatever the situation, there is only one solution to performance problems that arise from the mishandling of consequences by supervisors: The supervisors' behavior must change. This often begins when supervisors are made aware that they are a significant part of the problem—a difficult task, because it is typical for accused individuals to become hostile or defensive. However, if a supervisor is able to accept partial responsibility for the problem, it may then be necessary to help him or her learn new ways to deal with employees. An appropriate form of management training or informal coaching may be required.

THE INDIVIDUAL

Most organizations today expend great effort on selecting new employees, particularly at the management level. Every good recruiter knows that individuals are unique.

There is only one solution to performance problems that arise from the mishandling of consequences by supervisors: The supervisors' behavior must change.

Each person has certain physical, mental, and emotional qualities. Moreover, differ-

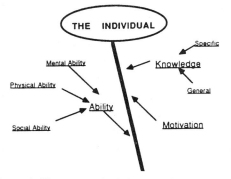

Figure 4. How well an individual performs on the job can be determined by mental and physical characteristics as well as by motivation and knowledge.

ent people are motivated by different things—some by money, some by hope of advancement, and some by a genuine desire to help people. Finally, the knowledge that a candidate brings to the job is critically important in a high-technology environment such as health care. All of these factors (summarized in Figure 4) are important in determining how well a person will perform on the job.

The most obvious type of individual "ability" is physical. Some jobs in health care require an employee to lift heavy loads. Others require the use of specific senses such as sight or hearing. It is entirely legal to refuse to hire people with certain types of handicaps for jobs in which they would be unsuccessful.

Less obvious as a job requirement is an individual's social ability. Many jobs in health care require what might be termed "emotional labor." As any nurse will testify, prolonged contact with people in physical and emotional need is hard work. There is a high rate of burnout among caregiving professionals.

By the same token, a position that requires high levels of public contact, such as that of a receptionist, also requires that the person hired to fill it has a certain level of "social stamina." People in high public contact positions need the ability to relate to patients and visitors in a uniformly helpful manner, often in very stressful situations. Although these public contact skills can be enhanced through training, personality factors have a far greater influence in determining how an employee will act on the job.

Perhaps the most difficult type of ability to judge is mental ability. Mental ability is most often equated with IQ. And yet, the term is also used to suggest an ability to exercise judgment and to see the potential implications of a course of action. Someone who makes a foolish mistake on the job is often accused of being "not too smart."

Effective selection procedures are the obvious starting point for improving the ability levels in an employee population. Years ago, certain testing procedures, including IQ tests, were used to screen applicants. Some of these tests have been ruled illegal and discriminatory by the courts. However, industrial and organizational psychologists have devised many other legally defensible methods for systematically improving the selection of employees. Assessment centers, although expensive and time-consuming, have been proven effective. Somewhat less expensive but also effective are behaviorally based interviewing techniques.[4]

Effective selection methods can also help in finding employees who can be motivated by the rewards offered by the organization. Generally, organizations can provide four types of reward: financial (money and job security), status (titles, a large office space, special parking), job content (creative job assignments, professional growth), and social (an opportunity to work with friends).[5] Although there is some controversy in academic circles as to whether money is a motivator, most experienced supervisors know that dollars can powerfully influence employee behavior.

However, it is also true that few people are motivated by money alone. The key to selection is identifying applicants who value the rewards available to a given organization. Thus a smaller hospital that cannot afford to pay top dollar for managerial talent might seek a candidate who, while willing to accept a fair wage, is motivated primarily by the desire to perform socially useful work or by the challenge of managing effectively.

Finally, every individual hired into an organization must at least possess a certain basic level of knowledge. It is not entirely clear to researchers what role knowledge plays in individual performance. The term "knowledge" is often associated with the educational system. However, educational level is not always the best predictor of performance. Almost everyone knows an employee such as the secretary who has only a high school education but who has been with the organization for years. Extensive knowledge of people and procedures makes this employee an invaluable resource to any department. The knowledge that makes this employee effective can be gained only through work experience.

In a sense, then, there are two types of knowledge—general and specific. General knowledge is usually gained in the education system. For example, an individual might learn the principles of budgeting in an undergraduate business program. Specific knowledge, on the other hand, is relevant only in a certain time and place. A general knowledge of budgeting does not mean that a new manager knows how to develop next year's budget in the organization he or she has just joined. Every organization has unique procedures that can be learned only through specific training or through on-the-job experience.

When it comes to knowledge, health care organizations face a "make-or-buy" decision. Highly trained professionals such as physicians, nurses, and therapists are usually hired with the knowledge required to do the job. In effect, the institution "buys" the knowledge that these professionals have gained through education. Unless the organization is a major teaching hospital, it is usually not cost-effective to train large numbers of these highly skilled employees. On the other hand, it may be entirely feasible to train less skilled clerical personnel and service workers internally.

FEEDBACK

It was noted earlier that information about the job comes from a variety of sources. Feedback is a special type of job information. Ideally, it is information that is received while the job is being done and that is used to guide the actions of the person doing

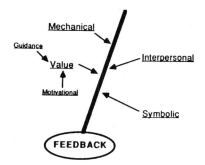

Figure 5. Information about a job comes from many sources, including feedback—information received on the job that guides the employee's actions.

the job. Figure 5 suggests that feedback may be mechanical (from the dial on a machine or the screen of a computer), symbolic (from the words and numbers on a printed report), or interpersonal (from peers and supervisors).

A good example of mechanical feedback is the information given by a car's speedometer. By watching the needle on the car's dash, a person can tell if the car is traveling within the posted speed limit. If the car is too fast, the speedometer "tells" the driver to slow down. If the car is too slow, then it lets the driver know when to speed up. In any case, a speedometer allows motorists to adjust their driving from moment to moment.

In the health care setting, feedback can come from a variety of sources. Most people are familiar with the simple dial on a blood pressure cuff. On a more sophisticated level, the computer screen of a diagnostic imaging unit allows the operator to make needed adjustments. Health care managers also depend on feedback from a variety of printed reports, of which the monthly budget report is a good example.

Feedback can also be interpersonal. People constantly look to others for information about how their actions affect them. Supervisors play an especially important role in giving interpersonal feedback. In their day-to-day contact with employees, supervisors constantly telegraph messages about whether they approve or disapprove of various actions. Wise employees watch these signals carefully.

All feedback has both a guidance and a motivational value. If feedback has an adequate guidance value, it will provide performers with information that allows them to correct their work performance on the

spot. To have this effect, feedback must be clear and understandable. Whether responding to the spoken word of a supervisor or to information on a budget report, performers must be able to translate messages into understandable terms so they can act on them.

Motivational value is most apparent in interpersonal feedback. Clear and unambiguous feedback coupled with positive reinforcement is one of the most powerful tools a supervisor has. Again, all people respond favorably to things they like, such as praise. When a supervisor states clearly what he or she likes about the employee's work performance, the employee understands better what is expected. Adding sincere praise to this feedback then increases the probability that the employee will continue to perform the desirable actions again. The art of positive reinforcement entails being clear and specific.

NO SIMPLE SOLUTIONS

Most work performance problems involve deficits in more than one of these major areas (inputs, consequences, feedback, or the individual). Thus, there is rarely a simple way to create a lasting solution to substandard work. It is a supervisor's responsibility, however, to look beyond "quick fix" solutions in order to create a work environment that is both efficient and effective.

In the case of our coding group, the consultant used the cause and effect diagram in Figure 1 to identify deficits in each of the following areas:

- *Workflow.* Because there was poor control of records between the time they left the nursing unit and were received by the coders, workflow to the group was uneven. The coders were either idle or overworked about 25% of the time.

- *Knowledge.* Training for the new coders was inadequate. New employees received a two-week orientation that involved reading a manual and working with an experienced coder. This type of training would be sufficient for less complex skills. However, the coding task called for more formalized training techniques.
- *Consequences.* The only consequences applied by supervisors to the coding group were negative. That is, whenever coders fell significantly below quality or productivity standards, they were "written up." Management in the department made little attempt to work with the coders individually or as a group to solve performance problems.
- *Feedback.* Individual coders had no way of keeping track of their own productivity on a regular basis. They usually found out they were performing below standard when the group's su-

pervisor called them in for a disciplinary session.

From this analysis, the consultant recommended a series of improvements that included the following:

- Tighter control of the workflow. This was the most critical improvement, because the group was literally unable to meet the department's productivity standards much of the time.
- An improved training program with a qualifying test that new coders must pass before joining the group.
- Development of a graphed-data feedback system to allow individual coders to monitor their own performance.
- Improved coaching by supervisory staff, with a major emphasis on positive reinforcement and positive discipline.

The result was that in six months the backlog disappeared entirely. Not one of the coders was fired, and morale in the group rose significantly. And finally, the director, because he had been flexible enough to follow the consultant's recommendations, received a significant pay increase for solving a problem that had cost the hospital over $1 million.

REFERENCES

1. Ishikawa, K. *Guide to Quality Control.* 2d revised ed. Hong Kong: Nordica International, 1982.
2. Bailey, R.W. *Human Performance Engineering: A Guide for Systems Designers.* Englewood Cliffs, N.J.: Prentice-Hall, 1981.
3. Vroom, V.H. *Work and Motivation.* New York: Wiley, 1964.
4. Byham, W.C. "Toward a Content-Valid Personnel System." In *Virginia Tech Symposium on Applied Behavioral Science. Vol. 1,* edited by J.A. Sgro. Washington, D.C.: Heath, 1981.
5. Sink, D.S. *Productivity Management: Planning Measurement and Evaluation. Control and Improvement.* New York: Wiley, 1985.

Revising the production process: when "more" is not the solution

Karen Zander
Organizational Development
Specialist
Department of Nursing
New England Medical Center
Boston, Massachusetts

ALTHOUGH THE HEALTH care world is rapidly changing, many managers feel that the important aspects of their work do not change fast enough. They and their staff come to work ready to do battle[1] daily, struggling with dysfunctional work designs, poor management information systems and outdated, constraining policies. Even with the best personnel, work that could otherwise be readily accomplished requires monumental struggle.

Chronicity—a term long used to describe certain patients' health status—also describes the nature and duration of problems afflicting many health care institutions. These problems are felt most acutely by frontline workers and their immediate managers. The consequences, translated into expense, errors and frustration, also are being felt acutely by health care administrators.

The times are ripe for change, and

Health Care Superv, 1985,3(3),44–54

the health care supervisor is in a key position to provide critical information to administration about the nature of current problems and their possible resolution. An ability to use a social–technical–environmental (STE) approach to the production process over which the health care supervisor has jurisdiction will establish the supervisor as a valuable internal consultant for the consideration of necessary large-system changes.

THE MIDDLE MANAGER'S CHANGING ROLE: DREAMER TO ANALYST

The fantasy

Middle managers in health care can be characterized as harboring a sustaining fantasy: "If I could just have more people to do the work, the work would be easier, my people would be happier and I could feel satisfied." Until recently, the manager's role was largely seen as protecting turf, enforcing interturf policies and occasionally making well-timed, heartfelt bids for more people and equipment. For instance, the solution to nursing care delivery problems was perceived to be more staff; the solution to drug distribution was perceived to be satellite pharmacies and unit dose delivery systems; the solution to covering the expense of more equipment requested by physicians was to charge patients more money. In other words, pushing for more resources was acceptable

> *In other words, pushing for more resources was acceptable managerial behavior in most health care organizations.*

managerial behavior in most health care organizations.

Even before the current era of limited resources, "more" was not necessarily better; it simply provided the *image* of being better. For instance, the 1950s practice of two-week hospital stays for the postpartum period was not necessarily better, but it did often convey a sense of well-being and "good care." More people on a nursing staff budget gave the manager a false sense of security in filling out a time sheet, even if everyone knew that some of the staff would call in sick or be relatively nonfunctional even when they did show up as scheduled. Similarly, more committees and committee meetings left the institution with a sense that matters were being handled, even if committee time was wasted by late starts, unclear objectives and poor group-process facilitation.

Layering: a dysfunctional strategy

Along with the more–is–better philosophy in health care institutions came the phenomenon of layering: If one policy, procedure or department was not working, the institution would invent another layer of policy, procedure or personnel. Although appearing creative on the surface, upon closer inspection it can be seen that layering evolves from a sense of helplessness about making real change. As a result, the symptom rather than the disease is approached, and there is no resolution of the original difficulty.

An example of layering surfaced when it was learned that one medical center generated a high proportion of stat requests for laboratory work, an order theoretically reserved for the most critically ill patients. When most of the medical center patients had stat orders written—a practice later found to be reinforced by the fact that physicians were telephoned by the laboratory with results rather than having to look for the results on a clipboard—the laboratory and intensive care units invented a "super stat" category to indicate the *real* stats.

Another type of layering is the use of "new" categories of workers, such as physicians' assistants and licensed practical nurses (LPNs) to do professionals' work. It is common practice nationally to staff nursing units with a large percentage of LPNs although their salaries are not significantly lower than RNs and they cannot legally function within the broad scope of an RN. For a little more money or a slight change in staffing mix, RNs could perhaps provide more mileage under a particular state's nursing practice act. Instead of considering such options, however, many nursing departments struggle with the problems of how to make a place for LPNs in primary nursing or how to keep certain LPNs growing when they may have outgrown their roles. The same phenomenon can be seen with mental health workers in the psychiatric field.

One further example of layering can be seen in the duplication of work among various departments and disciplines. For instance, the admission procedure may be performed by at least three departments: admitting, physicians and nursing. How many times are patients asked about their allergies? How many times (and to whom) does a patient have to complain about an overstuffed wastebasket or a hard-boiled egg that was supposed to be soft-boiled? Much layering occurs when a department or discipline is not held accountable for its designated outcomes, and when the fear of mistakes (usually of omission) causes other segments of the institution to cover the same bases.

Parallel play and overcoming futility

In the past, managers had to rely on layering to maintain their own operations as each work unit went about its tasks in what one physician critically describes as "splendid isolation."[2] The way different departments carry out their operations is analogous to parallel play, when two or more children play at the same time in the same place but not together.

An example of parallel play can be seen in the practice of nursing making its case assignments (as in primary nursing) totally unrelated to who the physicians have in their caseloads. The result is built-in hurdles to effective collaboration so that even the most respectful of interdisciplinary clinicians have to remember, locate and communicate with an unmanageable number of people and variables.[3] With parallel play, the resources that are available fall victim either to underutilization or to the opposite, depletion.

The fantasy of more is better is persistent and pervasive, not because it works (if it comes true at all) but because it salves the sense of futility felt about any other change strategy. Health care supervisors need to believe that there are good reasons to dispel the myth and take an active role in helping their agencies provide high quality care using the same, fewer or different resources. "More is no longer better" summarizes Dr. Jerome Grossman, president of the New England Medical Center Hospitals in Boston.[4]

THE PRODUCTION PROCESS: KEY TO COST-EFFECTIVE CHANGE

Options to cutting costs

According to Peter VanEtten, chief financial officer of the New England Medical Center, there are six organizational approaches to cutting costs:[5]

1. "The Shotgun"—across-the-board percent cuts in staff or other resources;
2. "The Rifle"—cutting out the fat in specific services (IV teams, clinical specialists, etc.);
3. reducing services—eliminating the more vulnerable programs (i.e., health promotion, community outreach, research and teaching);
4. reducing quality—as in establishing quotas on orders for laboratory tests or X-rays, or decreasing the number of diapers used in pediatrics;
5. increasing volume—more surgical procedures; and
6. changing the production process—restructuring all aspects of delivering the product (practice patterns of professionals, information, technology, personnel utilization, etc.).

Of these six approaches, changing the production process is the most meaningful, but it is also the most complex. It provides a manager with maximum control in rethinking and implementing new systems that do not merely add to old ones but truly improve the way work is accomplished.

Analyzing the production process

Revising the production process entails analyzing three major subsystems over which the manager has jurisdiction: (1) social (the relationships that develop among the people doing the work); (2) environmental (formal groups external to the ones being studied that have an important bearing on the work flow); and (3) technical (what work is done and how it is accomplished). Hackman and Oldham state that: "While there are numerous useful system-oriented approaches to the analysis of work organization, [the Socio-Technical approach] stands out as having the most relevance to the design and redesign of jobs and work systems."[6]

An STE systems analysis is comprehensive (without being complicated), time-limited "action research." It possesses academic solidity and provides grassroots-generated assessment, problem identification and suggestions for resolution so that the manager can make highly informed decisions before making major changes.

IMPLEMENTING AN STE SYSTEMS ANALYSIS

Background

The STE systems analysis constitutes a framework for studying the three main components of a complex, continuous production process. It originated as Social-Technical system analysis during field work in 1951 in the coal-mining industry of Great Britain and continued in 1963 in a London metalworks factory. Because these studies revealed "striking evidence for the need to examine the relationship between the social and technological aspects of work as they relate to the environmental forces in the work situation,"[7] they can be applied to the health care delivery system.

The two known applications in health care were by students in 1974 at the Primary Care Center, University of California at Los Angeles Medical Center,[8] and in 1982–83 by the New England Medical Center's Management Project.[9] The Boston application has been refined in several ways, especially in formalizing the environmental segment of the analysis.

Rationale

The health care supervisor might have several purposes in mind for initiating an STE systems analysis. The most appropriate rationale would include getting at the heart of an issue that has interconnected, multiple causes by using a group of online workers to collaborate on all phases of investigation. It is appropriate in either a centralized or decentralized structure.

An STE systems analysis fosters self-reliance within the department by having a group study itself without undue interruption in the work flow.

An STE system analysis fosters self-reliance within the department by having a group study itself without undue interruption in the work flow.

It also goes beyond the opinion-oriented recommendations of quality circles because it generates hard data. The data are multiperspective in that the analysis does not focus exclusively on any one type of information (audit, time-study, etc.). Group implementation of the analysis coupled with the balanced categories of data fosters creative yet realistic recommendations that arise from a truly collaborative undertaking. The following list identifies the range of issues or questions about the production process that the health care supervisor might want addressed:

1. a specific issue or question, such as utilization of ancillary positions or orientation of new personnel;
2. a group of issues or questions, such as the effect of "flexitime" on costs and morale or the effectiveness of the discharge process between inpatient and outpatient departments;
3. a group of issues or questions facing a specific area as one of many interdependent groups in the health care system, such as the efficiency of the admitting process or the quality of information or teaching resulting from multidisciplinary rounds; and
4. a group of issues or questions shared by formal or informal multiprofessional groups within the organization, such as the productivity of a hospitalwide committee or the overlap and duplication of certain services.

Case application: Pratt 4

When the STE systems analysis was applied to Pratt 4, a surgical unit of the New England Medical Center, the purpose was to determine how the objectives of quality care, staff and patient satisfaction, and cost-effectiveness could be better met. A six-person action group of managers and staff was supported by administration for a two-month study of Pratt 4's production process. Examples of each of three STE components and the tools used to study them are included in Figure 1. This study was performed during work hours, which necessitated its completion in a short time-frame.

Highlights of a longer list of findings in each of the components demonstrate the various levels and also the common themes (layering, poor coordination and communications, etc.) of problems. Consistent with other applications of STE systems analysis, Pratt 4 used it to describe the intertwining of all aspects of the work "in rich and complete detail."[10]

Social analysis

The following were the findings from the social analysis:

1. Communications was identified as the number one area needing improvement. Physicians were frustrated because they often could not find the right primary nurse with whom to discuss a particular patient's care. Nurses wanted more discussion and planning for patient care with physicians. Technicians, aides and nurses sensed an unwritten rule against too much "upward communication"; rarely did they interact with physicians.

Components	Examples	Tools for Analysis
Technical System The work done and how it is accomplished	• Care of patient before and after surgery • Training of students • Assignments of workers • Flow of information • Geographic work flow	• A diagram of the floor's physical layout • A flow chart of a typical patient's progress through Pratt 4 • Industrial engineering time studies of a staff nurse, a secretary and a surgical intern
Social System The relationships that develop among the people doing the work	• Who frequently talks to whom • How disagreements are handled • Worker's perception of the work and each other's roles	• Interviews of 12 people in a wide variety of roles on the floor • Semistructured observations of people interacting on the floor
Environmental Systems Those units/groups external to the one(s) being studied that have an important bearing on its work flow	• Admitting, pharmacy, laboratories, social service, etc. • Nursing department beyond the area of study	• What services do they provide Pratt 4? • Who on Pratt 4 is the key contact to them? • What problems, if any, have developed? • How dependent is Pratt 4 on that service?

Figure 1. The STE systems analysis framework as applied to Pratt 4. Reprinted with permission from McCaskey, M. *A Framework for Organization Analysis: The Pratt 4 Project.* Watertown, Mass.: Cambridge Management Association, January 28, 1983.

Technical analysis

The following were the findings from the technical analysis:

2. Disagreement was often handled through passive avoidance. One person would demonstrate disagreement or displeasure by failing to respond to inquiries or suggestions from the other person. In addition, guilt was frequently employed, and a favorite ploy seemed to be to "put the monkey on someone else's back."

1. The discharge of patients is not well coordinated. These inefficiencies disrupt many other aspects of patient care, beginning with admission.

2. Nurses spend a lot of time traveling back and forth to the medication room, which is located at one end of the floor.

3. Interns, residents and attending physicians sometimes have to travel to more than ten floors to see their patients. Improving the discharge process would allow the admitting office to group

a physician's patients more closely together, thereby cutting down on travel time.

Environmental analysis

The following were the findings from the environmental analysis:

1. Because the discharge time is often vague and because transport personnel can suddenly show up to take a patient for tests, many meals are wasted. It is not possible to reheat a meal, so it is discarded.
2. The results of the environmental analysis posed a challenge for the action group because control over these issues was shared with other units of the hospital. In addition, the action group needed to work with the different services to jointly attack these problems.

The action group spent the greatest amount of time gathering facts, opinions and patterns, and in striving to see a larger picture before narrowing problems to one cause or source. In ten weekly two-hour meetings, brainstorming was balanced by attention to objectives and to remaining realistic. Symptoms were separated from underlying problems. Change proposals had to be directly related to cause and effect, but they also had to be flexible enough to be revised after further input (during the next phase of the project). In other words, the larger change proposals had to provide plenty of mileage, preserve the integrity of all interdependent groups

and lend themselves to quantification.

The group's eight change proposals are briefly described as follows:[11]

1. Increase communication between physicians and nurses at critical times (especially rounds) to better coordinate patient care.
2. Reallocate duties along with commensurate authority.
3. Establish collaborative practice among physicians, nurses and administrators via an ongoing management group.
4. Improve the discharge process by anticipating discharge dates and writing discharge orders the night before a day discharge.
5. Conduct a larger systems analysis of Pratt 4's interdependence with the laboratory, admitting office and pharmacy.
6. Institute standard orders for admission, beginning with the easier case types.
7. Exchange the location of the medication room with the more centrally situated coat room.
8. Reduce the number of wasted meals.

MANAGING CHANGES IN THE PRODUCTION PROCESS

Important considerations

After using STE systems analysis (or any other method of analysis) as a basis for change proposals, several crucial steps must be taken to manage the proposed changes in the production process. These steps are:

1. assigning responsibility to a person or persons to manage the changes;
2. assigning accountability to the same person or persons for the outcomes of the changes;
3. establishing times for formal evaluation of the outcomes of the changes against the baseline data and the original objectives;
4. ensuring support for the manager, who in turn must support the employees; and
5. developing mechanisms that will generate and evaluate new data about the production process.

Ongoing analysis and response

In the case of Pratt 4, a three-person group of managers called the DNA (for chief *d*octor, head *n*urse and unit coordinator, representing *a*dministration) was designated to implement the change proposals and further revise the production process. Since the first year after STE systems analysis, the DNA has met formally for one hour weekly to discuss current policies and practices on Pratt 4 and their relationship to costs. Some of this group's accomplishments have been:

1. Primary nursing case assignments have been realized for consistency with physician case assignments.
2. Nurse flexitime has been used to ensure that an RN is always on evening rounds. That nurse uses a list of the nonurgent requests of nursing staff for the day shift, which has drastically cut down on pages to physicians and has increased order writing.
3. Discharge orders and prescriptions written the night before discharge have been assured, which facilitates all other departments' abilities to accommodate patients.
4. The amount of patient waiting time from the admitting office to getting orders written has been reduced, partly through hospitalwide preadmission testing and also through the initiation of standard orders for commonly seen diagnoses. This speeds the production process for all departments that depend on those orders to begin service.
5. Discussions have been established between clinicians and nonclinical managers about quality, cost-effectiveness and the production process as it involves Pratt 4, pharmacy, the laboratories, computer users, social services, dietary depart-. ment, etc.
6. "Simple" changes have been instituted, like getting a microwave oven, transposing the location of the old medication room and the coat room, and changing the way nurses review medication sheets before administering drugs. These changes have seemed revolutionary and stimulating to the staff, and have concretely improved conditions for all involved.

With the original change proposals largely realized, administration has given its approval for the Pratt 4 DNA to extend its objectives into a new phase of change. Three major new goals involve more ways in which the productions process can be revised, supported and evaluated:[12]

1. Expand collaborative practice. As noted, this includes thorough review of the concept and implementation of an educational program for staff.

2. Review and attempt to utilize the data now being generated from case-mix and patient-acuity studies. The information gained should enable the DNA to look closely at practice patterns in order to identify areas in need of change.

3. Develop and implement methods of teaching efficient patient care in order to better contain costs. This process would include utilizing the information gained from the concurrent reporting system as well as the data generated from the case-mix and patient-acuity studies.

The DNA has found it to be true that "changes that are undertaken from a socio-technical perspective involve *simultaneous* modification of technical and social systems to create designs for work that can lead both to greater task productivity and to increased fulfillment for organization members."[13] Managing changes in production involves orchestrating the interdependencies of all special interest groups as they merge on a patient care unit.

In addition, the whole institution has come to see the Pratt 4 project as a microcosm of the problems and strategies that reflect the typical conditions in health care delivery. Over the past year, reporting structures and formal relationships between the surgical floor, the surgical department and the hospital as a whole have been clarified and augmented. Continued changes in the production process on Pratt 4 are linked to the way the entire surgical department functions, and in turn with the way the institution perceives and improves its operations. All levels of the organization are involved in better defining, understanding and creating accurate cost-related measures of change.

SUCCEEDING AT REDESIGNING WORK

Much of what happens in health care institutions is based on tradition. Until recently, institutions and their managers have had a stake in the status quo. Current cost-limiting legislation dictates that the values, principles, practices and processes of health care delivery must be reviewed and revised. Health care supervisors have the most significant role in work redesign.

To date the most comprehensive tool available to middle managers for the evaluation of the way work groups function is an STE systems analysis conducted at the unit level. An STE systems analysis allows the people who do the work to maintain control of what they do best as they gain a fresh view of that work. An STE systems analysis focuses on the production process, yet it includes the environmental contingencies of that process. Health care supervisors should adopt and adapt at least some aspects of STE systems analysis to gain objectivity, insight and effective approaches to their chronic troubles.

Having observed that "Middle managers assume a distant, 'wait and see' stance toward work redesign activities undertaken by their subordinate managers or by organizational consultants," Hackman and Oldham also state, "In our view, such a stance is ill-advised. For it is the behavior of middle managers, perhaps more than any other single factor, that ultimately determines whether work redesign turns out to be a success or yet another 'good idea that doesn't work in the real world'."[14]

VanEtten notes that "To reengineer a production process is to create a change in the culture of health care."[15] To even confront the status quo requires judgment, courage and commitment from the manager. In turn, the manager needs real support and responsiveness from administration. Together, they can create smooth production processes that do not sacrifice quality for cost.

REFERENCES

1. McCaskey, M. *A Framework for Organization Analysis: The Pratt 4 Project*. Watertown, Mass.: Cambridge Management Association, January 28, 1983, p. 7.
2. Cleveland, R. *The Pratt 4 Project*, video interview. Boston, Mass.: New England Medical Center, 1983.
3. Anderson, D., and Finn, M. "Collaborative Practice: Developing a Structure that Works." *Nursing Administration Quarterly* 8, no. 1 (Fall 1983): 19–25.
4. Grossman, J., *The Pratt 4 Project*.
5. VanEtten, P. "The Management Project," Presentation at the Nursing Management Forum, April 13, 1984, New England Medical Center, Boston, Mass.
6. Hackman, J.R., and Oldham, G. *Work Redesign*. Reading, Mass.: Addison-Wesley, 1980, p. 61.
7. Cummings, T., and Srivastra, S. *Management of Work: A Socio-Technical Systems Approach*. San Diego, Calif.: University Associates, 1981, p. 43.
8. Rogers, A., and Martini, M. "Socio-Technical Systems Analysis of the Primary Care Center." Unpublished manuscript, UCLA Medical Center, June 1974.
9. McCaskey, *A Framework for Organization Analysis: The Pratt 4 Project*, p. 4–9.
10. Hackman and Oldham, *Work Redesign*, p. 63.
11. McCaskey, *A Framework for Organization Analysis: The Pratt 4 Project*, p. 10.
12. Smith, T., Murphy, R., and Gunderson, R. "Pratt 4 Project Review." Memorandum, New England Medical Center, Boston, Mass. September 9, 1983, p. 7.
13. Hackman and Oldham, *Work Redesign*, p. 63.
14. Ibid., p. 157.
15. VanEtten, "The Management Project."

Productivity and the supervisor

John L. Templin, Jr.
Senior Director
Management and Planning
  Services
Hospital Association of New York
  State, Inc.
Albany, New York

IMAGINE YOU ARE a department head at Community General Hospital. You have barely enough time each day to get the work out, let alone to do some planning or finish next year's budget. Last week your administrator gave you a book to read, commenting that once you have read it, you will be able to motivate your staff to work smarter rather than harder. You wondered, though, whether administration realizes that your department is doing more work with less staff than it did last year; if only the book would tell you how to get administration to recognize the increase in work load.

Later that week you attended a special department head meeting called to discuss a new federal law and the potential impact it could have on the hospital budget. The administrator and fiscal director discussed the Tax Equity and Fiscal Responsibility Act of 1982 (HR 4691). "TEFRA," as they

Health Care Superv, 1983,1(3),1–11
© 1983 Aspen Publishers, Inc.

called it, was designed to create Medicare savings amounting to several billion dollars over the next three years. The savings will primarily be realized by cutting reimbursement to hospitals. Medicare will modify current reimbursement rules by establishing reimbursement ceilings for ancillary service departments, ranking hospitals according to case mix intensity, paying hospitals per admission rather than per diem, and perhaps placing Medicare under prospective reimbursement. The impact on your hospital could be substantially fewer dollars, which will translate directly into a smaller staff.

The administrator stressed that while there was no reason to panic the employees, it was vital to ensure that each department was as productive as possible. You were told that each department head should establish a mechanism to determine and monitor productivity. In the future, staffing decisions would be made only after presentation and evaluation of a documented need. You can understand the need to hold down hospital costs, but you now have more questions than answers. What is productivity? How is it measured? What is satisfactory productivity? How do you establish a staffing standard?

WHAT IS PRODUCTIVITY?

Most administrators are reasonable individuals and are looking for a fair day's work for a fair day's pay. What

constitutes a fair day's work? What is productivity and how much is enough? Productivity can be defined in many ways, but the simplest and most common definition is the ratio of "output" to "input." Output in health care facilities is measured in units of service or units of measure (e.g., patient days, laboratory tests, procedures, discharges, meals). Input is quantified in terms of employee time.

Productivity can be measured with either output or input being the numerator, depending primarily on the time it takes to complete one unit. In departments where the time per unit is more than one hour, the usual measure is hours per unit. In departments where the time per unit is one-half hour or less, the usual measure is units per hour. For example, in an inpatient nursing unit, productivity would be expressed as hours per patient day (HPPD), and the answer would be 4.0 to 20.0 HPPD or higher, depending on the type of unit. In a dietary department, productivity would be expressed as meals per hour (MPH). If the average time was 15 minutes per meal, the dietary productivity would be 4.0 MPH or 0.25 hours per meal. Either expression of productivity means the same, but one or the other may be easier to understand. The secret of productivity assessment lies in using standards and terms that you and your employees understand. While the dietary manager might understand either expression of productivity, few nurses or supervisors would understand nursing productivity if the standard was 0.05

> *The secret of productivity assessment lies in using standards and terms that you and your employees understand.*

patients per hour in an intensive care unit, or 0.25 patients per hour in a medical unit.

HOW IS PRODUCTIVITY MEASURED?

Units of measure

There are two primary units for measuring productivity: paid hours and worked hours. Paid hours encompass all paid time including regular hours, overtime hours, vacations, holidays, sick time and other paid time off (personal leave days, death in family, jury duty, etc.). Call-time hours are included only for hours paid when personnel are actually called in, and not for the shifts spent on call. Paid hours can be gathered from employee schedules, but the preferred source to ensure correctness and completeness is payroll reports. In gathering payroll data, overtime hours should be counted by clock hours even if paid at a premium rate of pay.

Worked hours are defined as only regular and overtime hours (including call hours when personnel are called in); vacations, holidays, sick time and other paid items off (VHS) are excluded. Two formulas can be used to determine productivity:

total units of service
$\div$ total hours = productivity
(units of service per hour)

total hours
$\div$ total units of service
= productivity
(hours per unit of service)

The first formula, resulting in units per hour, is commonly used in departments such as food service, laundry, laboratory or pharmacy. The second formula, resulting in hours per unit, is commonly used in nursing service, admitting or medical records. It is important to know which formula is being used for your department. If the "units-of-service-per-hour" formula is used, worked productivity is higher than paid productivity; if the "hours-per-unit-of-service" formula is used, paid productivity is higher.

In the first formula, for example, assume a dietary department in which there are 5,600 meals produced in two weeks, 1,400 worked hours and 1,520 paid hours; productivity is total units of service (meals) divided by total hours:

Worked productivity is 5,600 meals
$\div$ 1,400 worked hours = 4.00 MPH.

Paid productivity is 5,600 meals
$\div$ 1,520 paid hours = 3.68 MPH.

In this example, paid productivity is 8 percent lower than worked productivity.

In the second formula, for example, assume a medical/surgical nursing unit with 420 patient days in two weeks (30 patients per day), 2,100 worked hours and 2,320 paid hours. Productivity is total hours divided by total units (patient days):

Worked productivity is 2,100
  worked hours ÷ 420 patient days
                    = 5.00 HPPD.

Paid productivity is 2,320
  paid hours ÷ 420 patient days
                    = 5.52 HPPD.

In this example, paid productivity is 10.4 percent higher than worked productivity.

Setting a standard

Regardless of whether productivity is measured in units of service per hour or hours per unit of service, the resulting figure is meaningless unless you know what your productivity goal should be. You need a standard against which to compare your performance. That standard must be understandable and achievable. If the standard is 1.0 hours per unit and your department is producing at the rate of 1.1 hours per unit, you are using 10 percent more hours than the standard required to produce the volume of work. Conversely, if your department is producing at the rate of 0.9 hours per unit, you are using 10 percent fewer hours than the standard allows.

A standard should consist of the time required for a trained employee to produce one unit of output following approved methods while achieving an acceptable level of quality. It should not be set for either the best worker or the brand new employee.

If the work of a department tends to come in large batches for part of a day or for a few days of the week and at a lower rate at other times, the standard should represent an average situation. This adjustment to the average is particularly important in departments such as laboratories, medical records and admitting, and in nursing units such as intensive care units, operating rooms, delivery rooms and emergency rooms.

Management engineers express standards in one of three ways: (1) pure or normal, (2) standard and (3) target or performance goal. If you time an employee performing a function, and, on the average, the employee takes 1.0 hours to produce one unit, that is pure clock time or "normal" hours. It is recognized that the typical employee cannot continue producing at 1.0 hours per unit for the entire eight-hour paid workshift. The employee takes breaks, uses the bathroom, gets tired and gets interrupted. The management engineering phrase for these factors is personal, fatigue and delay time (PFD). If an employee is entitled to one 15-minute break and 20 minutes of additional personal time, the 35-minute total is approximately 7 percent of the eight-hour day. (If two 15-minute breaks are allowed, then personal time is 10 percent.) Typically, 5 percent factors are also added for fatigue and for minor delays, yielding a total PFD factor of 17 to 20 percent. Therefore, our 1.0 hour "pure" standard becomes a standard of 1.17 to 1.20 hours per unit.

Most hospital departments are not set up like factories. They do not have a backlog of orders, and they do not produce for inventory. You cannot hold requisitions for chest x-rays until you have sufficient volume to fully utilize the technologist, and you cannot perform three complete blood counts on a patient today rather than one today and one on each of the next two days. In addition, allowances must be made for orientation and training of new staff and continuing education of existing staff, for geographical layout or equipment problems, for fluctuations in volume and work mix and for standby capacity or minimum staffing coverage. The allowance is commonly called a target utilization or performance goal. It is expressed as a percentage or decimal and mathematically is used as a denominator. The factor should be established with management or with the assistance of a management engineer or consultant.

In the example above of a function taking 1.0 pure hours and 1.17 to 1.20 standard hours including PFD, a target can be set. If the PFD factor is 20 percent, then only 6.67 units can be produced in 8 hours ($8.0 \div 1.2 = 6.67$). If 6 units are produced, 7.2 hours will be utilized ($1.2 \times 6 = 7.2$) and 0.8 hours will be available for training or for standby (this example assumes that one employee completes the unit). If 7 units are produced, 8.4 hours will be utilized and 0.4 hours of overtime are likely. In this department, a 90 percent target utilization could be set so that the

time allowed for one unit becomes $1.2 \div 0.9 = 1.33$ hours. The time to produce 6 units now becomes 8.0 hours ($1.33 \times 6 = 8.0$) and the employee producing 6 units daily functions at target.

It is important to note in the foregoing example that the allowed time of 1.33 hours per unit is 33 percent more than the "pure" time of 1.0 hours as measured by time study. In departments with widely fluctuating work loads or large standby capacities (emergency rooms and delivery rooms), the target could be as low as 50 to 60 percent and the difference between the allowed time and pure time could be as much as 140 percent $[(1.2 \div 0.5 = 2.4) - 1.0] \div 1.0 \times 100$.

HOW DO YOU ESTABLISH A STAFFING STANDARD?

Setting a standard for variable work load

Standards can be set in many ways. The simplest method is a budgeted standard or "working at the same rate as last year." If your department is an ancillary service that produced 28,000 units in 1982 and if according to payroll reports there were 22,400 hours worked and 26,600 hours paid, and in 1983 you were budgeted for the same levels of volume and staffing, your standards would be determined by using formulas 1 and 2 in the boxed insert.

Suppose, however, that you were budgeting an increase to 30,000

Formulas for Determining Productivity Standards

(1) Worked productivity = 28,000 units ÷ 22,400 hours worked = 1.25 units per hour, or 22,400 hours ÷ 28,000 units = 0.8 hours per unit
(2) Paid productivity = 28,000 units ÷ 26,600 hours paid = 1.05 units per hour, or 26,600 hours ÷ 28,000 units = 0.95 hours per unit
(3) (14 FTEs × 2,080 hours per FTE) ÷ 30,000 units = 0.97 hours per unit or 1.03 units per hour

---

units, that you were authorized 14.0 paid full-time equivalents (FTEs) and your standard workweek was 40 hours. In this example, budgeted paid productivity would be determined by using formula 3 in the boxed insert. The standard was increased from 0.95 to 0.97 hours per unit, or approximately 2 percent.

What do you do when you are producing different units or if the time per unit varies significantly? If the units are of the same type but the time per unit varies as in a laboratory or in a radiology department, you develop a weighted average time per procedure. In the ancillary department discussed a few paragraphs ago, the following three procedures are performed:

Procedure A:	Volume,	9,000
Procedure B:	Volume,	10,000
Procedure C:	Volume,	9,000
Total	Volume,	28,000

If you are setting a budgeted standard and if volume is increasing uniformly, it does not matter how long each of the three procedures takes.

Suppose, however, that procedure A is being replaced by procedure C

for many patients and that the time per occurrence is significantly different. Now you must begin to set an "engineered standard." You time study the three procedures and find that procedure A takes 30 minutes, B takes 45 minutes and C takes 40 minutes. The calculations for the past year are shown in Table 1.

The average procedure took 38.57 minutes or 0.64 hours. If you determined that a 20 percent PFD factor was appropriate, the standard would be 0.64 × 1.2 = 0.77 hours per unit. Since the department actually worked at 0.80 hours per unit, it functioned at 0.77 required ÷ 0.80 actual = 0.96 or 96 percent target utilization.

The expected volumes and calculation of standards for the current year differ from those for the previous year (see Table 1). The average procedure will take 39.50 minutes or 0.66 hours. If you still use a 20 percent PFD factor, the new standard will be 0.66 × 1.2 = 0.79 hours per unit. Applying the 96 percent target utilization means that the department should function at 0.82 hours per unit (0.79 ÷ 0.96 = 0.82). This is an increase in standard of approximately 2 percent

Table 1. Calculations for determining average time per procedure

	Volume	Standard	Total minutes
Calculations for past year			
Procedure A	9,000	30.00	270,000
Procedure B	10,000	45.00	450,000
Procedure C	9,000	40.00	360,000
Total	28,000	38.57	1,080,000
Calculations for current year			
Procedure A	7,000	30.00	210,000
Procedure B	11,000	45.00	495,000
Procedure C	12,000	40.00	480,000
Total	30,000	39.50	1,185,000

and would correspond with the new budget of 14 paid FTEs.

Some departments' work load varies according to two factors; therefore, a two-part variable is necessary. For instance, the variables for a business office or a medical record department could be both discharges and outpatient visits. One variable could drop at a time during the year when the other variable is increasing.

> *Some departments' work load varies according to two factors; therefore, a two-part variable is necessary when establishing a standard for measuring productivity.*

Setting a standard for nonvariable work load

In the foregoing examples, it was assumed that there were three differ-ent procedures performed and that all work associated with them was variable. In many departments, part or most of the work load is not variable. The management engineering term used is *constant hours*. Examples of constant hours are many management functions, secretarial functions, supply functions, monthly report functions and cleaning functions. If in the example department there is one department head who is a "nonworking" supervisor and a secretary not included in the variable standard, the paid productivity for last year would still be 0.95 hours per visit, but it could be expressed as a constant plus a variable as follows: constant of 2.0 paid FTEs + [(26,000 − 4,160 paid hours) ÷ 28,000 units] = 0.80 paid hours per unit. Now if volume increased to 30,000 units but the mix stayed the same, the required paid hours would be: 4,160 hours + (30,000 units × 0.80 paid hours per unit) = 4,160 + 24,000 = 28,160 paid hours.

The new paid productivity would be 28,160 hours ÷ 30,000 units = 0.94 hours per unit. This is 0.01 hours per unit less than the productivity previously determined when all hours were treated as being variable. As a rule of thumb, when productivity is expressed as hours per unit and when there is a constant as part of the standard, if volume increases, the overall productivity standard decreases; if volume decreases, the overall productivity standard increases.

There are many types of constant functions. Some common examples are education of others, orientation of new employees, research and development, meetings, coverage during lunch and breaks for other employees and terminal cleanup. Time expended for some of these activities varies, but the basis for change is some factor *other* than the work load units being measured. For example, time spent in orientation of new employees varies more because of turnover rate rather than work load volume changes.

The most common way of expressing the constant in a productivity formula is to convert the time to a per-calendar-day basis. In the example above, the 4,160 hours per year for the department head and secretary converts to 11.40 paid hours per calendar day. This may be confusing if the department functions only five days per week, or if the individuals treated as constant work only weekdays, but it makes for a simple productivity formula: 11.40 paid hours per calendar day + 0.80 paid hours per unit. The formula becomes important when monitoring performance over time and in converting to FTEs.

Why FTEs?

As shown above in developing the staffing standards for the department with three procedures, the numbers can get large in a hurry. For management purposes, smaller numbers are much easier to understand. The time required last year to produce 28,000 units was 1,080,000 minutes. Who can comprehend one million minutes? When the time is converted to 18,000 hours, it begins to be understandable. Most supervisors know that one full-time employee is paid approximately 2,000 hours per year; therefore, at least a staff of nine is needed. The reader will recall that the department head had to add a 20 percent PFD factor and apply a target utilization of 96 percent, so the required worked staff was about 11 FTEs. Eleven is a number we can all understand. Full-time employees normally work five shifts per week.

By definition, an FTE is any full-time employee. An FTE is also any combination of part-time or per diem employees totaling five shifts per week. The number of shifts is more important than the shift length. Most hospital employees work an eight-hour paid shift. For them, one FTE is 40 hours per week or 2,080 hours per year (40 hours per week × 52 weeks per year). In some hospitals, the workshift is 7.5 hours so that one FTE is 37.5 hours per week or 1,950 hours per year. In a few hospitals, the workshift is only 7 hours so that one FTE is 35 hours per week or only 1,820 hours per year. In any hospital the workshift is the hours paid, not the hours between starting and leaving. If an employee reports at 8:00 A.M., leaves at 4:30 P.M. and has an unpaid 30-minute lunch period, the paid workshift is 8 hours.

The length of the workshift or the annual hours per FTE become important when hiring or when making multihospital comparisons. Depending on the length of the workweek, in a department with 26,600 paid hours, the numbers of FTEs would vary as follows: *40-hour week:* 26,600 hr. ÷ 2,080 hr. per FTE = 12.8 FTEs; *37.5-hour week:* 26,600 hr. ÷ 1,950 hr. per FTE = 13.6 FTEs; *35-hour week:* 26,600 hr. ÷ 1,820 hr. per FTE = 14.6 FTEs.

It is easy to see why a union would push for a shorter workweek—dues are collected on a per-employee basis. Expand this example from a department to an entire hospital or medical center and the difference can be 100 employees or more for the same total hours paid.

Many hospitals are introducing variations on the traditional 5-day, 8-hour workweek, particularly in response to nurses who are asking for flexible work hours. Common examples are the 4-day, 10-hour workweek and the 3-day, 12-hour workweek. For determination of FTEs, these hospitals still rely on the standard definition of 40 hours per week or 2,080 hours per year.

Why both worked and paid productivity?

The example used above was a department with 22,400 worked hours and 26,600 paid hours. Assuming a 40-hour workweek, the department had 10.8 worked FTEs (22,400 ÷ 2,080) and 12.8 paid FTEs (26,600 ÷ 2,080). The difference of 2.0 FTEs reflects employees on vacation, holiday, sick time and other paid time off (VHS). The 2.0 FTEs can be expressed either as a percentage of worked or paid FTEs. When building a budget from standards and volume (zero-based budgeting), it is necessary to calculate a percentage to be added to worked FTEs as a "markup." In the example, the markup is 18.5 percent (2.0 ÷ 10.8 × 100). The VHS as a percentage of paid staff is a "markdown" of 15.6 percent (2.0 ÷ 12.8 × 100). In budgeting, it is essential to know which approach was used to develop the VHS percentage. Using the wrong approach for this department would yield an error of 2.9 percent or 0.3 FTEs. Extending the error to the entire hospital would yield a difference of many FTEs which could lead to serious financial or personnel problems.

What should VHS be?

Last year the VHS was 2.0 FTEs in the department. Was that good or bad? How can you tell? The first step is to convert the VHS percentage to paid days off per FTE and then to compare the answer with the days off per FTE allowed by the personnel policy with the actual use rate in other departments. The conversion is accomplished in one of two ways, either of which yields the same result. A paid FTE is paid for 52 weeks × 5 days per week or 260 days per year. If the VHS is used as a percentage of paid time, the paid days off are simply 260 × VHS markdown percentage or 260 × .156 = 40.6 days per FTE. If the VHS is used as a percentage of worked time, the paid days off are 260 paid days − 260 ÷ [paid FTE (1.0) + VHS markup] or 260 − [260 ÷ 1.185] = 260 − 219.4 = 40.6 days per FTE. The 219.4 in the second method is the worked days per FTE per year.

The 40.6 VHS days per FTE could be 20 days vacation, 10 holidays, 10 sick days and 0.6 days of other paid time off. If your payroll system captures sufficient detail, you should analyze the components for your department and determine if they are reasonable. For instance, if new employees receive two weeks vacation to start, three weeks after five years and four weeks after ten years, unless all of your employees have ten years' service with the hospital, an average of 20 days vacation is impossible. A more plausible answer may be that sick days were 15 days per employee because one or two long-term employees were out for extended periods because of major illnesses or accidents. In such a situation, it is less

likely that the same thing will happen during the coming year, and you should budget using a lower VHS percentage.

There is another fairly common reason for a given cost center to have an unusually high VHS factor, particularly if similar cost centers at the hospital have lower factors—employees may be pulled or "floated" from the cost center because of peaks elsewhere or drops in work load in the home cost center. It could be that the cost center is a medical/surgical nursing unit closed several weeks for renovation or because of an extended drop in volume. In such situations, the worked hours may get credited to other cost centers, yet the entire VHS stays in this cost center. The result is that there appears to be a high VHS factor when in truth the factor was inflated because the VHS hours were not floated out.

WHAT IS ACCEPTABLE PERFORMANCE?

A department may expend exactly the budgeted hours per year and may achieve exactly the budgeted volume, but doing both is highly unusual. Many factors affect the staff level, for example, resignations and replacement problems, random sick calls and major illnesses and variations in workload throughout the year. Although, on an annual basis, the budgeted volume might be achieved, month-to-month swings of 20 to 30 percent are common. In resort areas, work load indicators such as emergency room visits may double or triple during busy months.

Recommended ranges of performance are necessary on both a monthly and a year-to-date basis. In any given month, productivity should fall within plus or minus 5 percent for proper staffing and within plus or minus 10 percent to be within acceptable limits. If the department is over- or understaffed between 5 percent and 10 percent, it bears watching; if it is more than 10 percent over- or understaffed, management attention is indicated.

Recommended ranges of performance are necessary on both a monthly and a year-to-date basis.

On a year-to-date basis the variances should be smaller, since the peaks and valleys tend to cancel each other. To be considered properly staffed, a department's productivity should be within plus or minus 2 percent, and to be within acceptable lim-

its, productivity should vary no more than plus or minus 5 percent. If a department remains outside a corridor of plus or minus 5 percent for several months, management action is indicated. As a word of caution, in sections or departments with less than 10 FTEs, small FTE variances convert into large percentage variances. Instead of percent ranges, use plus or minus 0.5 FTE as the acceptable range for both monthly and year-to-date productivity variances.

●　　●　　●

Productivity has always been important in hospitals. With the advent of TEFRA it becomes even more important. The goal of each manager must be to produce more output for the same or less input. Therefore, managers must be able to explain productivity to their superiors and subordinates, be able to set productivity standards and project staffing requirements. Once productivity is within an acceptable range it must be monitored to ensure that it stays within range.

Productivity monitoring for every supervisor

John L. Templin, Jr.
Director
Productivity Improvement Division
Applied Leadership Technologies,
Inc.
Greenfield Center, New York

NO MATTER what magazine one may pick up, whether health care journal or general interest publication such as *Newsweek*, it is not possible to read many pages without coming across some reference to the need to "be more productive" in order to survive in today's economy. It seems that no longer is anyone talking about "quality care." What is the meaning of this change for the health care supervisor? How do the supervisor's interests and needs compare with those of the other key players on the management team—the administrator, the fiscal director and the personnel director? Does it seem as though the administrator is interested only in keeping the medical staff and board happy, that the fiscal director is interested only in the bottom line, and that the personnel director is interested only in keeping the employees from joining a union or from going on strike? Are productivity

Health Care Superv, 1984,2(4),35–47
© 1984 Aspen Publishers, Inc.

measurement, improvement and monitoring specialized or difficult processes requiring outside resources, or can the supervisor pursue them personally? Should one reinvent the wheel for the thousandth time, or are there readily available methodologies and tools that can fill the bill and allow the supervisor to make more effective use of limited time? All of these are valid questions deserving the health care supervisor's close attention.

THE CHANGE IN EMPHASIS

Why the sudden emphasis on productivity? Hospitals do not simply add or retain staff just to have more than the hospital down the street or across town. Administrators and department heads have always recognized that there is a cost associated with staff. Until the start of hospital fiscal years beginning October 1, 1983, and later, hospitals in much of the country were paid on the basis of charges or on a retrospectively determined per-diem rate. Under this reimbursement system it was easy to retain staff who were no longer productive, and it was easier to add personnel rather than capital equipment that required certificate-of-need (CON) approval. There was little incentive to contain costs.

Nationally, Medicare paid about 36 percent of the hospital costs. In individual hospitals, the Medicare portion was frequently 50 to 60 percent.

The federal trust funds for Medicare were rapidly being depleted and would soon be bankrupt if the rate of increase of costs could not be controlled.

In September 1982, Congress passed legislation requiring hospitals to be paid for care provided to Medicare patients on the basis of prospectively determined costs per discharge with the costs being grouped by diagnosis related groups (DRGs). Hospitals were told that they would be paid fixed rates per DRG and that if the cost of care was more, the hospital would have to reduce costs or bear the loss themselves. Conversely, if the care could be provided less expensively, the facility could keep the "profit." As a result, hospital boards, administrators and fiscal directors began to talk of productivity measurement, improvement and monitoring. New buzz-words came forth, including cost per discharge (rather than per-diem costs) and product-line costing (rather than cost per unit of service).

PRODUCTIVITY REVIEWED

Productivity is defined as the ratio of output to input (refer to "Productivity and the Supervisor," HCS 1:3, April 1983). Output in health care facilities is measured in units of service (e.g., patient days, discharges, laboratory tests, procedures, meals). Input is quantified in terms of employee time. The most common expressions of productivity are "units per hour" (e.g., meals per hour, College of American Pathologists workload units per hour), or "hours per unit" (e.g., nursing hours per patient day, hours per discharge). In either expression, the hours can be paid hours or worked hours. Paid hours encompass all paid time including regular hours, overtime hours, vacations, holidays, sick time and other paid time off. Worked hours are defined as only regular and overtime hours.

Productivity standards

Productivity becomes important only once a goal is established and actual productivity is compared with that goal. The standard must be understandable and achievable. It

---

Productivity becomes important only once a goal is established and actual productivity is compared with that goal. The standard must be understandable and achievable.

---

should consist of the time required for a trained employee to produce one unit of output following approved methods while achieving an acceptable level of quality. It should not be set for either the best worker or the brand new employee. The standard should include an allowance for personal, fatigue and delay time (PFD).

Since most hospital departments are not set up like factories, do not have a backlog of orders and do not produce for inventory, allowances must also be made for fluctuations in workload and for standby capacity. Frequently called a *target utilization* or a *performance goal*, the allowance is normally expressed as a percentage. A 90 percent target would mean that ten hours must be worked to produce nine hours of quantified activity. Frequently the target will include allowances for orientation and training of new staff, for continuing education of existing staff, for geographical layout or equipment problems and for minimum staffing coverage.

Standards can be set in many ways. The simplest method is a budgeted standard or "working at the same rate as last year." Simply divide the total workload units by the total worked or paid hours to get budgeted units per hour. This assumes that the entire workload is variable. If the department is producing different units or if the time per unit varies significantly, a weighted average time per unit can be developed. In some departments, the workload varies according to two factors; therefore, a two-part variable is necessary when establishing a standard for measuring productivity. In many departments, part or most of the workload is not variable. This part of the workload is called "constant hours." Examples include management and secretarial functions, supply functions and monthly report functions. An example of a variable standard is 5.4 hours per patient day for a medical nursing unit. An example of a mixed standard is 5.0 hours per patient day plus 13.7 hours per calendar day for head nurse and unit clerk. If the average daily census is 34 patients, either formula yields the same staffing requirement. For higher census levels the full variable formula yields a higher requirement and for lower census levels the mixed formula yields higher staffing requirements.

What is acceptable performance?

While a department may expend exactly the budgeted hours per year and may achieve exactly the budgeted volume, accomplishing both is highly unusual. Many factors affect the staff level, including resignations, replacement problems, sick calls and major illnesses. Workload may vary during the year or in total, either due to changing medical staff membership or, as is being seen in many parts of the country, due to DRG reimbursement changing medical practice patterns. Recommended ranges of performance are necessary on both a period and a year-to-date basis. In any given period, productivity should fall within plus or minus 5 percent for proper staffing and within plus or minus 10 percent to be within acceptable limits. On a year-to-date basis, the variances should be smaller, since peaks and valleys tend to cancel each other. To be properly staffed, a department's productivity should be within plus or minus 2 percent; to be within acceptable limits, productivity should vary no more than plus or minus 5 percent.

HOW SHOULD PRODUCTIVITY BE MONITORED?

Assume that standards have been set for the department and that the supervisor and administration agree on the total projected workload and authorized staffing levels. The fiscal director has cooperated in quantifying the payroll costs including differentials, and the personnel director has worked out a plan to recruit for newly authorized or vacant positions. Now what? What can and should the supervisor do at the operating level to monitor productivity so as to avoid being surprised by the monthly budget reports and avoid getting well into the fiscal year only to be requested to lay off staff to balance the budget?

First, one should try not to panic. The supervisor is not alone; every manager in the facility has a need to monitor productivity. Second, one should ask questions. Is there a corporate plan for productivity monitoring, or does the organization participate in a regional or national productivity monitoring system? What are administration and the other managers doing? Third, if necessary, one can develop a customized monitoring system. It is not difficult to do; someone with access to a microcomputer can write a monitoring program in a couple of hours. It can also be accomplished manually with little more effort. Manual methods usually take less time to establish initially, but may require more time per reporting period to do the calculations. Manual methods are also more prone to error.

What is needed?

To monitor productivity, certain information is required. The six key elements are budgeted and actual volume, actual worked hours or full-time equivalents (FTEs), budgeted and actual paid hours or FTEs, and the productivity standards. The budgeted volume and budgeted paid hours usually need to be gathered only once per year, and standards need be audited or updated only once each year. The actual volume, worked hours and paid hours must be gathered each period the report is generated. One word of caution: one must be certain that the budgeted levels used are the same as the levels that administration and finance are using. It is not unusual for budgets to get changed during the budgetary approval process without department heads knowing about the changes until the first variance reports arrive and they are called to task for unacceptable performance. Also, one must be certain that the actual volume used in the report agrees with the volume administration or finance uses in their reports. For example, nursing may monitor using the 7 A.M. census level, only to learn that finance is using the

midnight census and that one-day stays and same-day expirations are being handled differently.

How to read a productivity monitoring report

The best way to explain how to read a report is by using an example. Figure 1 is a sample biweekly productivity report of a medical nursing unit. The budgeted volume level is 458 patients per two weeks or 32.7 patients per day. The unit is monitored biweekly immediately after payroll data are available. The report was set up on a microcomputer using a spreadsheet package; strange numbers appear for the last six cycles because no data are shown. The budgeted vacation, holiday and sick time factor used was 13.9 percent. The budgeted levels were developed as follows: 458 patient days times a standard of 5.49 hours per patient day equals 2,514 hours per two weeks; 2,514 hours divided by 80 hours per FTE equals 31.4 required worked FTEs; 31.4 times 1.139 vacation, holiday and sick time (VHS) factor equals 35.8 paid FTEs.

For the two weeks ending January 9th, actual volume was 485 patient days. Dividing 485 by 14 days yields 34.64 patients per day (actual volume was higher than budgeted volume). The actual manhours per unit of service (MH/US) was 5.29 or 0.20 less than the standard. The 5.29 MH/US is calculated by dividing the actual 2,568 worked hours by the actual 485 patient days. The standard of 5.49

GENERAL HOSPITAL
PRODUCTIVITY MONITORING REPORT

DEPARTMENT: MEDICAL   BUDGETED VOLUME: 458 PATIENTS PER 14 DAYS

PERIOD ENDING	ACT. VOL.	DAILY VOL.	REQ'D MH/US	ACT. MH/US	WORKED FTE'S REQ'D	FTE'S ACTUAL	VARIANCE FTE'S	VARIANCE %	PAID FTE'S BUDGET	PAID FTE'S ACTUAL	VARIANCE FTE'S	VARIANCE %	VHS %	WORK HOURS	PAID HOURS
01/09	485	34.64	5.49	5.29	33.3	32.1	-1.2	-3.6	35.8	40.6	4.8	13.3	26.4	2568	3245
01/23	495	35.36	5.49	5.47	34.0	33.8	-0.1	-0.4	35.8	36.6	0.8	2.3	8.3	2707	2931
02/06	503	35.93	5.49	5.34	34.5	33.6	-0.9	-2.7	35.8	39.3	3.5	9.7	16.9	2686	3141
02/20	490	35.00	5.49	5.43	33.6	33.3	-0.4	-1.0	35.8	38.2	2.4	6.6	14.7	2662	3053
03/06	492	35.14	5.49	5.58	33.8	34.3	0.6	1.7	35.8	37.4	1.6	4.3	8.8	2747	2988
03/20	487	34.79	5.49	5.61	33.4	34.2	0.7	2.2	35.8	37.0	1.2	3.3	8.2	2733	2958
04/03	455	32.50	5.49	6.08	31.2	34.6	3.4	10.8	35.8	38.8	3.0	8.5	12.3	2767	3107
04/17	431	30.79	5.49	6.29	29.6	33.9	4.3	14.6	35.8	38.0	2.2	6.0	12.0	2712	3037
05/01	486	34.71	5.49	5.64	33.4	34.3	0.9	2.8	35.8	37.1	1.3	3.5	8.1	2743	2965
05/15	486	34.71	5.49	5.52	33.4	33.5	0.2	0.6	35.8	37.2	1.4	3.9	10.9	2683	2976
05/29	476	34.00	5.49	5.47	32.7	32.5	-0.1	-0.4	35.8	37.4	1.6	4.5	15.1	2602	2994
06/12	500	35.71	5.49	5.29	34.3	33.0	-1.3	-3.7	35.8	39.6	3.8	10.7	20.0	2643	3171
06/26	500	35.71	5.49	5.57	34.3	34.8	0.5	1.5	35.8	36.9	1.1	3.1	6.0	2786	2954
07/10	445	31.79	5.49	6.05	30.5	33.7	3.1	10.2	35.8	40.5	4.7	13.2	20.5	2692	3243
07/24	449	32.07	5.49	5.96	30.8	33.5	2.7	8.6	35.8	39.9	4.1	11.5	19.2	2678	3193
08/07	392	28.00	5.49	6.81	26.9	33.4	6.5	24.0	35.8	37.6	1.8	4.9	12.6	2669	3004
08/21	426	30.43	5.49	6.11	29.2	32.5	3.3	11.3	35.8	35.9	0.1	0.2	10.3	2602	2871
09/04	451	32.21	5.49	5.78	30.9	32.6	1.6	5.2	35.8	36.9	1.1	2.9	13.2	2605	2948
09/18	451	32.21	5.49	5.65	30.9	31.9	0.9	2.9	35.8	35.7	-0.1	-0.3	12.0	2549	2855
10/02	428	30.57	5.49	5.80	29.4	31.1	1.7	5.7	35.8	34.8	-1.0	-2.9	12.0	2484	2782
10/16		0.00	5.49	ERR	0.0	0.0	0.0	ERR		0.0	0.0	ERR	ERR		
10/30		0.00	5.49	ERR	0.0	0.0	0.0	ERR		0.0	0.0	ERR	ERR		
11/13		0.00	5.49	ERR	0.0	0.0	0.0	ERR		0.0	0.0	ERR	ERR		
11/27		0.00	5.49	ERR	0.0	0.0	0.0	ERR		0.0	0.0	ERR	ERR		
12/11		0.00	5.49	ERR	0.0	0.0	0.0	ERR		0.0	0.0	ERR	ERR		
12/25		0.00	5.49	ERR	0.0	0.0	0.0	ERR		0.0	0.0	ERR	ERR		
Y.T.D.	9328	33.31	5.49	5.74	32.0	33.3	1.3	4.1	35.8	37.8	2.0	5.5	13.3	53318	60416

Figure 1. General hospital productivity monitoring sheet.

hours per patient day times 485 patient days then divided by 80 hours per FTE yields 33.3 required worked FTEs. This is 1.2 FTE more than the actual 32.1 FTEs (2,568 worked hours/80 hours per FTE). The 1.2 FTE variance is 3.6 percent. Actual paid hours were 3,245 so that actual paid FTEs was 3,245/80 or 40.6. This was 4.8 paid FTEs, or 13.3 percent, over budget. The VHS percent was 3,245 paid hours minus 2,568 worked hours or 677 divided by 2,568 worked hours yielding 26.4 percent.

This was an interesting two weeks, in which the unit had slightly more than budgeted volume (about 6 percent), worked with 3.6 percent less staff on duty than required and simultaneously was 13.3 percent over budget due to using 8.5 FTEs of vacation, holiday and sick time. This is a position many department heads have found themselves in; they expected a drop in volume during the holidays and scheduled staff vacations to use authorized time off. However, actual volume was higher than expected and other staff had to be brought in and overtime had to be used to provide appropriate on-duty coverage. The result was that the unit operated over the paid budget.

By reviewing each of the 20 cycles and the year-to-date (YTD) rows, one can see how the cost center functioned. The year-to-date average volume was 0.6 patients per day higher than budgeted, worked FTEs showed 1.3 higher than required, paid FTEs showed 2.0 higher than required, and the vacation, holiday and sick time used was 0.6 percent less than budgeted.

This is one example of an internally generated monitoring report. Supervisors should experiment with developing their own reports or consider adapting the report shown in Figure 1 for their own use. In doing so, it is important to remember that if part of the productivity standard is a constant, the required MH/US will vary slightly inversely to volume changes. If a supervisor does not feel

---

It is important to remember that if part of the productivity standard is a constant, the required manhours per unit of service will vary slightly inversely to volume changes.

---

comfortable developing a reporting system, or if the hospital is using an external system, the supervisor should learn what data are fed into the system, should gain access to the reports and should learn how to read the reports.

EXTERNAL MONITORING SYSTEMS

Monitrend

The oldest and best known monitoring system is a service of the American Hospital Association (AHA) called "Monitrend." When the service was first released it was referred to as the "Has" Reports or Hospital Administration Services Reports.

Monitrend is a fee-for-service product subscribed to by more than 2,500 hospitals nationally. Each month the facilities complete an input form containing statistical, financial and staffing data. The data are computer processed and comparative reports are produced showing how each hospital performed relative to other hospitals in the same group. Groups are normally hospitals in national, state and regional bed-size ranges plus many special groups that a hospital may request. Monitrend also offers a comparison of facilities with similar medicare case mix indices based on DRGs as assigned by the health care finance administration.

The Monitrend monthly reports consist of 29 pages including executive, nursing services, ancillary services, support services, raw data and data audit sections. Until 1983 the reports were all based on paid hours per unit of service. Reports are now also available showing worked hours per unit of service. Individual department standards are not part of Monitrend; the comparisons are of a hospital's hours per unit of service to the group median and quartiles. A sample page from a Monitrend report is shown as Figure 2. The page is 24, "Laundry & Linen and Dietary Services."

Each page is split into a comparison with group median data and an internal trend data section. The dietary group median data show that for the prior three months this hospital's total meals per patient day of 4.87 is slightly below the national median of 5.00 for 246 reporting hospitals and slightly above the state median of 4.78 meals per patient day. The 3.03 patient meals per patient day is in the fourth quartile for both comparisons. The direct expense is only 3.43 percent of total hospital cost, which compares very well nationally and is in the bottom 5 percent in the state. The paid hours per 100 meals of 23.39 also is in the first quartile for both groups. The extension on the far right shows that the hospital used 9.05 hours per 100 meals fewer than the national average, and that converts into 1,203 hours fewer for the month based on total reported volume. If one divides by 173 hours per FTE per month, the difference is 7.0 FTEs less than the median hospital. The internal trend data show that the dietary results have stayed about the same for the last 24 months.

Resource Monitoring System

Another service, which has been available for more than ten years, is the Resource Monitoring System (RMS) offered by the Hospital Association of New York State. RMS differs from Monitrend in that the reports do not compare one hospital's performance with a group of hospitals but rather with engineered standards established specifically for the facility. RMS has always used the difference between required and actual worked staff hours rather than paid staff hours as the basis of comparison. One reason for choosing worked hours is that the VHS add-on percentage in New

Monitrend II Hospital Report with Worked Hours—Level 3
Support Services—Group Data

Laundry & linen	Hospital indicator	Ind Qtr	Ind Qtr	Ind Qtr	Ind Qtr	Code	Variance	Multiplier Value	Extention
Total pounds per patient day	26.74	19.59 4	24.50 3	25.66 3	20.99 3	A			
Contract pounds per patient day									
Total direct expense per 100 lbs.	36.29	34.19 3	34.04 3	38.47 2	32.77 3	B			
Inhouse direct expense per 100 lbs.	36.29	25.34 4	21.86 H	26.45 4	28.36 4	B			
Inhouse salary expense per 100 lbs.	27.51	18.14 4	16.02 H	18.15 H	18.41 3	B			
Inhouse ODE per 100 lbs.	8.78	6.06 3	6.32 H	7.33 4	8.12 3	B			
Contract expense per 100 lbs									
Inhouse PUR service expense percent salaries									
Total laundry direct expense percent	0.88	0.83 3	0.72 H	0.75 3	0.81 3				
Revenue per calendar day									
Worked hours per 100 lbs.	3.38	1.25 4	1.50 H	1.45 H	2.30 4	A			
PCT worked hours to paid hours	86.99	90.28 2	91.64 1	91.53 1	89.96 1				
Inhouse average hourly salary	7.08	6.50 3	6.51 3	6.57 3	6.38 3	B			
Paid hours per 100 lbs.	3.89	2.90 4	2.13 H	2.65 4	3.09 4	A			

Support Services—Internal trend data
(raw data represent the numerator used to calculate indicators in first 2 columns)

Laundry & linen	June 1990	3 months ending May 1990	3 months ending May 1989	Percent change	3 months ending May 1988	Percent change	Current month	Prior 3 month average	Description
Total pounds per patient day	26.00	26.74	25.32	5.61	26.08	2.53	13026	18397	POUNDS
Contract pounds per patient day									CTR-LBS
Total direct expense per 100 lbs.	38.93	36.29	34.95	3.83	35.13	3.30	5071	6676	DIR-EXP
Inhouse direct expense per 100 lbs.	38.93	36.29	34.95	3.83	35.13	3.30	5071	6676	DIR-EXP
Inhouse salary expense per 100 lbs.	34.16	27.51	28.56	-3.68	25.20	9.17	4449	5061	SAL-EXP
Inhouse ODE per 100 lbs.	4.78	8.78	6.39	37.40	9.93	-11.58	622	1615	ODE
Contract expense per 100 lbs.									DIR-EXP
Inhouse PUR SVC EXP % salaries									
Total laundry direct expense percent	0.63	0.88	0.91	-3.30	1.06	-16.98	5071	6676	
Revenue per calendar day									REVENUE
Worked hours per 100 lbs.	3.89	3.38	4.11	-17.76			507	622	WKD-HRS
PCT worked hours to paid hours	79.84	86.99	97.40	-10.69			507	622	
Inhouse average hourly salary	7.01	7.08	6.76	4.73	6.56	7.93	4449	5061	SALARIES
Paid hours per 100 lbs.	4.88	3.89	4.22	-7.82	3.85	1.04	635	715	PD-HRS

A=National-50 through 74 beds; B=Oregon-50 through 99 beds; C=Oregon-all bed sizes; D=R6-<100 beds, CMI: 1.120+

Figure 2. Sample page of AHA Monitrend II™ report. Reprinted with permission from American Hospital Association, Chicago, Ill., 1990.

York State hospitals ranges from 12 to 20 percent. An 8 percent difference between staffing levels for similar departments in two hospitals could be significant or could simply be due to differences in paid time off. There are also large ranges in most other states. As part of any productivity monitoring activity, supervisors should always check to see what the VHS percentage is in their departments and in similar departments of other hospitals in the same region or state.

RMS reports are generated on the cycle chosen by the hospital, either every four weeks or every month. There are two types of reports per cycle: an Administrative Report showing how all the cost centers fared against their standards, and Trend Reports for each cost center. The Trend Reports show individual department performance for the period and for year-to-date. A sample Administrative Report is shown in Figure 3.

Other monitoring systems

Several other organizations offer productivity monitoring systems. The acknowledged first system was CASH-LPC, the labor performance control system (LPC) of the Commission on Administrative Services to Hospitals (CASH) developed in California in the 1960s. Current systems with general acceptance include CHI Management Information System (CHIMIS), the management information system of Chi Systems, Inc.; Productivity Monitoring Program (PMP),

which replaced Total Labor Control (TLC), as the system of the Ohio Hospitals Management Services; Productivity Audit and Review, CHHS (PAR-C), the system of Sun Alliance, formerly the Carolinas Hospitals' Shared Services; plus systems internal to several of the for-profit hospital chains. (No endorsement of any system is intended. The foregoing list is not meant to be all-inclusive but is presented simply to provide examples of systems a manager might encounter.)

HOW TO USE A MONITORING REPORT

Developing a productivity monitoring report or receiving a periodic copy of a report on the performance of one's department is not the final step. Rather, it is but one step on the road to productivity improvement. Productivity improvement is not a program to be introduced, serve a finite useful life and then be scrapped. Productivity improvement should become an integral part of the management process and should be ingrained in staff at all levels from the chief executive officer to the newest worker at the lowest salary grade. If top management and management staff members at all levels are committed to it, productivity will improve.

The two-edged sword

Too often, productivity studies are undertaken with the specific goal of reducing staff in a department or

Page __1__ of __4__   Period Ending: 4/30/82   Run Date: 6/22/82

DEPARTMENT	UNIT OF SERVICE	UNIT OF SERVICE ANALYSIS					PRODUCTIVITY ANALYSIS					BUDGET ANALYSIS				
		Budgeted Volume	Actual Volume	Daily Volume	Variance %	Actual MH/US	Required FTE	Actual FTE	Variance FTE	Variance %	Variance Prior 3 Periods	Budgeted FTE	Actual FTE	Variance FTE	Variance %	Variance Yr. To Date
2A M/S	PATIENT DAYS	810	782	26.1	-3	4.66	20.6	22.2	-1.6	-8	-7	26.3	25.1	1.2	5	4
2C M/S	PATIENT DAYS	725	698	23.3	-4	4.48	16.4	18.3	0.1	1	10	23.2	19.3	3.9	17	16
2CX M/S	PATIENT DAYS	660	686	22.9	1	4.50	18.1	18.1	0.0	0	-7	22.2	19.9	2.3	10	5
3A M/S	PATIENT DAYS	825	841	28.0	2	4.78	22.2	23.5	-1.3	-6	-4	23.7	25.4	-1.7	-7	-9
3B & 3E M/S	PATIENT DAYS	1405	1189	39.6	-15	4.90	31.4	34.1	-2.7	-9	-1	29.6	37.4	-7.8	-26	-36
3C M/S	PATIENT DAYS	935	901	30.0	-4	4.84	23.8	25.5	-1.7	-7	-9	32.2	29.0	3.2	10	8
4E M/S	PATIENT DAYS	320	469	15.6	47	5.31	12.4	14.6	-2.2	-18	-10	24.3	15.9	8.4	35	36
MED/SURG SUBT	PATIENT DAYS	5700	5566	185.5	-2	4.80	146.9	156.3	-9.4	-6	-4	181.5	172.0	9.5	5	3

Figure 3. Sample administrative report, Resource Monitoring System. Reprinted with permission from CHART, Inc., Albany, New York.

throughout an entire hospital. Most multidepartment studies show that there are cost centers with more staff than required, some with proper staffing and some that are understaffed. If management is committed to cutting staff, it must also be committed to adding staff in those cost centers where more people are needed. A too large staff leads to excessive cost, poor work habits and the potential for error and low morale. A too small staff can lead to the better workers leaving to go to organizations in which they can practice their skills effectively, to increased malpractice claim exposure and to poor morale or union overtures.

Productivity monitoring reports should be used for both short-term planning and long-range planning. In the short term, they should be used as guides for determining when to replace staff, to put a temporary hold on new hiring, to readjust daily staffing patterns, to transfer staff from one cost center to another, to encourage vacations and other paid time off and to allow or forbid the use of overtime. In the long term, they should be used for annual budgeting, vacation planning, scheduling special projects or renovations, and (as they are increasingly being used), as part of the basis for management compensation. Nonprofit hospitals as well as for-profit hospitals are turning to incentive-based compensation for department heads. One basis for a bonus at the end of the year is productivity improvement. The improvement can consist of either more efficiently us-

ing the existing resources or developing and implementing more efficient and cost-effective systems.

Staff involvement

The day when the manager was assumed to be the only person with the facts and figures, and the brains to use them, and when staff members were assumed to be unwilling to share in responsibility has gone. Theory X management rarely works today. Quality of work life (QWL) and quality circle (QC) programs are flourishing. Cost center managers must work to ensure that their staffs understand the basis for standard setting, the process for calculating the required staffing levels and the contents of monitoring reports. If a cost center has a trend report showing performance relative to goals, the report should be shared with the staff. The periodic results should be reviewed and the staff should participate in productivity improvement studies. The productivity monitoring report should be posted in a place readily accessible to the staff and staff members should be encouraged to read the report and voice any questions they may have. While cost reduction is a byproduct of the system, the main reason for productivity mon-

The main reason for productivity monitoring is to ensure that quality patient care continues to be available at a reasonable cost.

itoring is to ensure that quality patient care continues to be available at
a reasonable cost.

PARTING THOUGHTS

One does not need a microcomputer, a degree in management engineering or computer science or a
large staff to get involved in productivity monitoring and productivity
improvement. Any cost center manager with a $10 calculator, knowledge
of the department and the desire to
succeed *can* succeed. One can set
productivity standards based on the
units of service produced, and can
talk to peers in other facilities to find
out how others are doing. It is possible to know approximately how well
one's cost center performed even before the report comes out, and one
should be able to explain why there
are variances.

Good productivity is a result of
continuous hard work. If the cost center shows understaffing, it is due to
handling increased volume with the
same staff or handling the same volume with less staff input. If overstaffing is the case, the opposite applies.
One cannot always predict what will
happen to volume or staffing, but
one's management worth can be revealed by the manner of reacting to
what does happen and how well one
plans to avoid the same things happening again in the future. It may not
be possible to stay within plus or minus 5 percent every period, but it is
possible to work with upper management and with one's own staff to assure that the cost center's average
productivity and staffing stay within
the limit. With DRG reimbursement
and with an increasing number of
professionals competing for decreasing numbers of management positions available, if one cannot or will
not control and improve productivity
there will be many who will gladly
take over the task.

The impact of nonwidget-producing activities

John L. Templin, Jr.
President
Templin Management Associates,
Inc.
Greenfield Center, New York

WIDGET IS A slang term for gadget. It has been used to describe a product in many fields. Gadgets can be very simple or extremely complex. To produce a widget one must follow the steps in a procedure. The cost of the widget will consist of the direct labor and supply cost plus overhead for other essential activities at the widget plant. There will be accounting, clerical, and supervisory costs in addition to costs for orienting and training the widget makers.

In health care the product is the improved health of a discharged patient, within, it is hoped, the approved diagnosis related group (DRG) length of stay. The cost of improved health will be the direct labor and supply cost plus overhead for other essential activities in the department and hospital.

In hospital departments the product or output is expressed in various terms, such as patient days, tests, pro-

Health Care Superv, 1987, 5(4), 13–26
© 1987 Aspen Publishers, Inc.

cedures, meals, or discharges. Productivity is defined as the ratio of output to input.[1,2] Managers in most U.S. hospitals have seen the output, or units of service, decrease during the past few years. Admissions are down slightly, patient days are down dramatically, and some nursing units have closed. The federal government has tightened up on reimbursement and is expected to tighten more in order to achieve a balanced budget.

Hospital administrators have responded to reductions in volume and revenue by reducing staffing, either by not replacing staff who leave or by layoffs and other forced moves. Most commonly, the staff reductions occur at the rank-and-file, or production, level with little or no impact on management or staff positions. This article discusses the impact of staffing reductions on the paid staffing requirement and the impact of activities (e.g., supervision, clerical support, and supply functions) related to the production of work on the staffing requirement of any department.

THE IMPACT ON PAID TIME OFF

Employee turnover occurs most rapidly during the first year of employment; the turnover rate decreases with increasing years of service. There are many reasons for this. During the probationary period, typically 60 to 90 days, employees who are not working out can be terminated with little or no problem. Union contracts allow for such termi-

nation, and government agencies usually do not interfere with such decisions. Employees during their first three months of employment normally are not entitled to use vacation time, and if they cease employment they are not compensated for unused time. The same is true for paid sick days. During the probationary period many hospitals also restrict the use of holidays and, particularly, personal leave days.

When an employee leaves with less than one year of service, it is common for no vacation time to be paid. Employees with more than one year of service but less than five years typically receive fewer paid vacation days per year than employees with more service. An example of a vacation policy is two weeks of vacation for more than one year but less than five years of service; three weeks of vacation for five years but less than ten years of service; and four weeks of vacation for ten or more years of service. If staff are not replaced when they leave, the average seniority creeps up for the remaining employees, as a higher percentage becomes eligible for the increased vacation entitlement.

Staffing reductions because of layoff are usually based on seniority; the persons with the least seniority are the first laid off. If there is a recall, the persons with the most seniority are the first recalled. Therefore, when a layoff occurs the average paid days off per year for the remaining employees increase. For example, as shown in Table 1, if paid staff were

Table 1. Analysis of the impact of staffing reductions on available staff

Position	Initial FTEs*	Prereduction staff		10% staff reduction			10% salary reduction		
		Days off per year	Worked FTEs	Paid FTEs	Days off per year	Worked FTEs	Paid FTEs	Days off per year	Worked FTEs
Manager	1	43	.83	1	43	.83	1	43	.83
Assistant Manager	1	43	.83	1	43	.83	1	43	.83
Section Head	6	43	5.01	6	43	5.01	6	43	5.01
Assistant Section Head	6	41	5.05	6	41	5.05	6	41	5.05
Medical Technician 3	12	40	10.15	12	40	10.15	12	40	10.15
Medical Technician 2	20	39	17.00	20	39	17.00	20	39	17.00
Medical Technician 1	25	30	22.12	19.6	30	17.34	17.8	30	15.75
Secretary	2	40	1.69	2	40	1.69	2	40	1.69
Clerical 2	2	36	1.72	2	36	1.72	2	36	1.72
Clerical 1	4	30	3.54	3	30	2.65	2	30	1.77
Phlebotomist	4	28	3.57	2	28	1.78	2	28	1.78
Diener	1	40	.85	1	40	.85	1	40	.85
Total	84.0	36.0	72.4	75.6	36.7	64.9	72.8	37	62.4
Percent paid days off		13.85			14.12			14.22	
Staffing change percent				10		10.29	13.33		13.71

* Full-time equivalents.

As shown in the column labelled 10% staff reduction, if paid staffing is cut by 10%, worked staffing is cut by 10.29% since the remaining employees average an extra .7 paid days off per year. As shown in the column labelled 10% salary reduction, in order to reduce salaries by 10%, paid staffing must be reduced by 13.33% and worked staffing by 13.71% since the remaining employees average 1 extra paid day off per year compared to the original staffing level. These are sample data for illustration only.

Reprinted with permission from Templin Management Associates, Inc.

reduced by 10 percent, the staff available for work would be reduced by approximately 10.3 percent. The impact could be even greater if the staff that were eliminated were entitled to less vacation. For instance, if nursing was cut 10 percent by eliminating some aides and by totally eliminating the evening shift clerical coverage, and if these employee groups received two weeks of vacation to start while new registered nurses (RNs) started at four weeks of vacation, the staff available for work could be reduced by 11 to 12 percent, because the number of paid days off increases. The same situation could occur in a laboratory, pharmacy, or any department with a mix of professional and support personnel. The important effect to remember in any downward staffing adjustment is the impact on staff available for work.

CREATING MORE WORKED TIME

Typical expressions of productivity are hours per patient day, hours per test, or hours per 100 College of American Pathologists (CAP) workload units. Improvements in productivity are expressed as reduced hours per unit of service. In the previous example, if volume decreased by 10 percent and paid staff also decreased by 10 percent, the paid hours per unit of service do not change. The worked hours per unit of service drop slightly, and there may be the perception of improved productivity. Conversely, if it is necessary to work

at the same productivity rate as prior to the reduction, either volume will have to drop more than 10 percent or paid staffing will drop by less than 10 percent. It may be that the additional hours are worked as overtime hours at a cost of time-and-a-half, which will drive up the cost per unit of service. Incidentally, the cost per unit has undoubtedly increased since the staff eliminated were paid a lower hourly rate of pay. In other words, to cut 10 percent in salary costs a manager may have to cut the number of employees by 12 to 15 percent. This is illustrated in Table 2 where a staff reduction of 10 percent results in a salary cost reduction of only 7.5 percent. In order to achieve a 10 percent reduction in salary costs, paid staffing must be reduced by 13.3 percent. As shown in Table 1, due to a higher percentage of paid time off for the remaining staff, overall worked staff available is cut by 13.7 percent.

If there is fat in the system, some can be eliminated. This could mean less standby or idle time, a slightly longer time for response or service, or fewer hours of coverage. For example, when a patient must be transported, the patient may have to wait an extra few minutes to be transported. A department may eliminate routine service on the evening shift after 8:00 P.M.

Improvements can occur in other ways. A new piece of equipment with faster throughput time or better on-line recording and transmission of results can improve productivity, provided that the hours made available

Table 2. Analysis of the impact of salaries on staffing reductions

Position	Average salaries		Prereduction staff		10% staff reduction*		10% salary reduction	
	Annual	Hourly	FTEs	Annual $	FTEs	Annual $	FTEs	Annual $
Manager	$50,000	$24.04	1	$50,000	1	$50,000	1	$50,000
Assistant Manager	$40,000	$19.23	1	$40,000	1	$40,000	1	$40,000
Section Head	$35,000	$16.83	6	$210,000	6	$210,000	6	$210,000
Assistant Section Head	$31,000	$14.90	6	$186,000	6	$186,000	6	$186,000
Medical Technician 3	$27,000	$12.98	12	$324,000	12	$324,000	12	$324,000
Medical Technician 2	$24,000	$11.54	20	$480,000	20	$480,000	20	$480,000
Medical Technician 1	$21,000	$10.10	25	$525,000	19.6	$411,600	17.8	$373,800
Secretary	$20,700	$9.95	2	$41,400	2	$41,400	2	$41,400
Clerical 2	$15,600	$7.50	2	$31,200	2	$31,200	2	$31,200
Clerical 1	$13,000	$6.25	4	$52,000	3	$39,000	2	$26,000
Phlebotomist	$11,960	$5.75	4	$47,840	2	$23,920	2	$23,920
Diener	$21,840	$10.50	1	$21,840	1	$21,840	1	$21,840
Total	$23,920	$11.50	84	$2,009,280	75.6	$1,858,960	72.8	$1,808,160
Percent change					10	7.48	13.33	10.01
Average hourly salary		$11.50		$11.50		$11.82		$11.94

* Full-time equivalents.

As shown in the column labelled 10% staff reduction, if staffing is cut by 10%, the salary cost is only cut by 7.48% since the personnel eliminated are at a lower annual salary. As shown in the column labelled 10% salary reduction, in order to reduce salaries by 10%, staffing must be reduced by 13.33%. In actual practice, the salary cost per FTE within grade will increase due to the fact that new employees are usually paid a smaller salary. The new average hourly rate is $11.82 in the 10% cut in FTEs and $11.94 in the 10% cut in costs. These are sample data for illustration only.

Reprinted with permission from Templin Management Associates, Inc.

are no longer worked. Systems and procedures can be streamlined, or the department can perform more work with the same staff. (However, work is not increasing in most hospitals.)

Management engineers typically express the required staffing level for a department as a formula:

worked hours (WH) =

$$\frac{(\text{var} \times \text{vol} + \text{con} \times \text{days})}{\text{target utilization (TU)}}$$

The variable (var) is the variable standard per unit of service such as hours per test. Volume (vol) is the number of units of service produced during the time frame. Constant (con) is the amount of time required per day for those functions that either are fixed (constant) or vary based on a factor other than the primary volume. Days is the number of days in the time frame such as 14 days (biweekly) or 365 days (yearly). The target utilization (TU) is a factor to allow for standby and idle time plus other unmeasured activities.[3]

The College of American Pathologists has done an outstanding job of recognizing and quantifying constant activities. The *CAP Manual on Workload Recording* refers to this component of work as "nonworkloaded" activities.[4] Seventeen separate categories are listed in the 1987 CAP manual, and Appendix 3 explains each in detail. Although appearing in a laboratory publication, the categories of constant activity apply to most departments in virtually every health care facility. These activities are legitimate and necessary to support the main purpose of the department. However, the amount and variation in the required amount of time is largely independent of the variation in the primary workload indicator. For this reason, the constant activities can be reviewed and changed as necessary to improve productivity.

Constant activities can be reviewed and changed as necessary to improve productivity.

Two examples may help clarify the difference between variable and constant activities. The first example concerns the two cleaning activities in an operating room: cleaning after each case and cleaning at the end of the daily elective schedule. Cleaning after each case varies somewhat based on the type of surgery, but a common time frame is 15 minutes per case. If two cases are performed in the room on a given day, then 30 minutes of cleaning time are required. If six cases are performed, 90 minutes of cleaning time are required. Since the time per case is constant but the total time per day varies with the number of cases, after-case cleanup is normally a variable activity. Terminal cleanup at the end of the day frequently takes 30 minutes per room; this is a fixed time whether two cases or six cases were performed in the room. The total time per day varies based on the number of rooms used rather than on the number of cases per room. Thus, it is expressed as a constant of 30 minutes per room per day.

Another example is the cashier function. The time required for each transaction at the window is approximately the same or can be averaged. The total time is dependent on the number of transactions and can be expressed as a time per transaction, such as 1.5 minutes per transaction. If 200 transactions occur in a shift, the total time required is 300 minutes (5 hours). The time to cash out and take the receipts to the bank or other repository is fixed or approximately the same each day. Thus, the total time varies based on the number of times per day or per week that the cashier cashes out or takes receipts to a bank.

Methods improvement studies can lead to reduced time per room for cleanup or reduced time per cashier transaction. Room utilization studies can lead to fewer operating rooms being scheduled on a given day. These improvements result in a lower variable standard per unit of service.

The remainder of this article will concentrate on identifying the variety of constant activities, quantifying the time expended on these activities, and discussing ways to reduce or eliminate the time.

CONSTANT ACTIVITIES

Accounting, billing, and related activities

Accounting, billing, and related activities occur in many departments. On a nursing unit these functions in-

clude the time to prepare and deliver requisitions or charge slips. In ancillary departments they include time for processing of the requisition and batch preparation and delivery of slips to the business office or other department.

Administrative and supervisory time

Administrative and supervisory time varies primarily based on the number of employees, style of management, skill level of employees, and turnover rates rather than being directly related to the variable workload. A food service department with 20 employees each working a four-hour evening shift requires more supervision than a food service department with 10 employees each working an eight-hour shift, even though the total hours worked per day are the same.

Administrative activities include budgeting, recruiting, orienting new staff, counseling, disciplining, doing performance appraisals, scheduling employees, reading mail, performing professional society functions, attending informal meetings, preparing management reports, and the like. Often overlooked is the time spent by employees receiving counseling, disciplinary action, and performance appraisals.

There is no correct or single answer as to how much supervision is enough. Titles can be misleading. There are departments where 15 percent to 20 percent of the staff have titles that suggest management or supervisory positions. Many of these individuals are "working supervisors" who spend very little time managing. Typical examples are charge nurses or assistant head nurses, section heads or assistant section heads in laboratories, and persons in many departments with the term "senior" in their job title. An extreme example encountered was "lead diener" in a two-person autopsy section in a teaching hospital laboratory. The lead diener spent one hour per week attending a management meeting; therefore, 2.5 percent of his time and 1.25 percent of the total time for the section was supervision. A typical percentage of total staff time in a cost center for management or supervisory functions is 4 percent to 10 percent, depending on the nature of the cost center. Most commonly it is 5 percent to 7 percent.

Breaks and personal time

As discussed in the CAP manual, breaks and time for personal necessities are sometimes treated as a constant activity. More commonly they are a percent add-on to the variable staffing standard. Whichever way this activity is handled, it is a significant portion of the staffing equation. If one break per employee per day is allowed, it is about 3.5 percent of total worked staffing, and if two breaks per employee per day are allowed, it is 7 percent of total worked staffing. When breaks are treated as a constant, be sure to count the employees only on the days they are physically present in the department. If full-time employees have 30 paid days off per year, they can take breaks only during the 230 days they are working.

Clerical support to management and other staff

Clerical support should be only that portion of the clerical person's worked time that is not spent producing part of the variable workload. For example, in a diagnostic imaging department (radiology) the time to type the report is generally considered part of the variable standard. Clerical support includes handling and distributing mail, photocopying, typing letters and administrative reports or procedures, screening telephone calls, working on payroll, setting up meetings, and typing minutes. Clerical support is frequently 2 percent to 4 percent of total staffing.

Computer activities

With the introduction of microcomputers and word processing in many hospital departments, computer activities can be time consuming. This includes systems analysis, programming, editing of computer files, database management, investigation of system malfunctions, and other related functions. There are other computer-related activities that are generally recognized as part of the variable standard including initial entry of test requests or results.

Courier activities

A common complaint in nursing is that an aide or unit secretary is frequently off the unit running for supplies or carrying requisitions. A medical records department may send a clerk to each nursing unit to collect the charts for patients discharged the previous day. An electrocardiogram (ECG) department may send a clerk to each nursing unit with the ECG reports. Courier activities also include the time spent picking up specimens drawn by other staff.

It may be possible to reduce the time spent by assigning the work to a small group of staff or by consolidating trips. If each nursing unit sends a report to the nursing office at the end of each shift, one unit secretary can stop at each unit rather than many persons making the trip. Perhaps the reports can be dropped off on the way home by an employee so that the time is cut in half since there is no return trip to the nursing unit. On the other hand, if unit staff remain on the unit and the work is assumed by others, is the time really saved? Departmental staff satisfaction or medical staff satisfaction may improve, but if eight unit secretaries each spend one hour per shift on errands and this work is now taken over by one messenger, did the hospital add the messenger and still pay for the eight secretaries, or was overtime reduced?

Educational activities

As the federal government changes how medical education is funded, educational activities are receiving close scrutiny in many institutions. Educational activities include both formal programs and support to programs. In some hospitals, the educational staff or coordinator are in a separate cost center; in the same department of another institution the persons may be in the primary cost center. Examples include schools of radiologic and medical technology. These may be either separate departments or part of radiology or the clinical laboratory. When making multihospital comparisons, it is essential to know whether the other hospitals have educational programs and how the staff are reported.

In addition to the program coordinator of full-time instructor, management or staff in the main department may also be involved in educational activities. Laboratory section heads may spend several hundred hours per year preparing lectures, setting up classrooms, giving lectures or exams, and correcting exams. Bench technologists may spend time with students at the bench, drawing station, or bedside. If this activity is present and is being quantified, only the additional time required for teaching should be counted, not the total time spent with students. For example, if four hours are used to do work that would have taken three hours if students were not present, only one hour should be counted for education.

Another potential source for double counting the time for education is when a resident or intern is working with a manager or supervisor and the manager's time has totally been accounted for as administrative activity. Counting several hours per week spent with the intern in addition to administrative time results in overstating the total time.

Housekeeping/infection control

Staff in many departments routinely spend time on housekeeping and infection control without that time being recognized or allowed for. This includes cleaning and disinfecting refrigerators, medical equipment, bench tops, and supply areas. This could also include an annual purge of old files.

Inservice or continuing education

Inservice and continuing education could include both inside and outside programs, depending on the payroll system. In many institutions, time spent at seminars or outside programs is recorded on the payroll system as "other" and does not appear as worked hours. Instead, it is lumped with the variety of nonworked paid hours such as vacation, holiday, sick time, and other paid but not worked time (e.g., bereavement leave). If this is the case, the worked hours will be slightly reduced as compared to other institutions, and the use rate of paid time off will be slightly higher. This method is typically used only for full day programs rather than short outside meetings.

Inservice within the institution varies by facility, department, skill level, and shift. Managers in many professional and technical departments desire one hour of inservice or continuing education for each professional or technical employee per month. This is .7 percent of the worked staff time. Occasionally, a department may provide the staff with one hour of education per employee per week. However, given cost constraints this practice is being questioned by administrators. Ancillary and clerical staff typically do not receive inservice at the same rate as professional or technical staff. A common rate is one hour every two or three months depending on the nature of the department.

Ideally, inservice should be available to all staff regardless of when they work. In practice, however, inservice is most commonly available on the day shift and primarily only on weekdays. Evening, night, or weekend staff may not receive inservice other than mandatory programs such as fire and safety or cardiopulmonary resuscitation.

Part-time and per diem staff pose another problem. Given the fact that most health care workers have every other weekend off if they are required to work weekends, many departments rely heavily on part-time or per diem staff for weekend coverage. Since these individuals work fewer days per year to maintain their skills, it could be argued that they require more inservice education than the full-time staff. If part-time personnel receive the same one hour of inservice per employee per month, however, a department with part-time staff will spend more hours and a greater percentage of total hours on inservice. For example, if one nursing unit has 20 full-time staff and each attends one hour of inservice per month, the total time is 240 hours per year. If another unit has 13 full-time staff and 14 part-time staff, each averaging half time, there would be the same 20 full-time equivalents (FTEs), but there would be 27 hours of inservice per month and 324 hours per year. This is an increase of 84 hours worked per year per unit that, if extended to all nursing units in a medium or large hospital, could equal at least one FTE or approximately $25,000 per year.

Repairs and maintenance

In some departments, routine daily or periodic repair and maintenance may be built into the variable staffing standards. Such is the case in the laboratory. In many other departments, this time plus the time for emergency repairs must be estimated and allowed for. For example, computerized tomography (CT) units are routinely scheduled for maintenance one-half day per week or per two weeks depending on the unit and its rate of use. If the staff or management participate in diagnosing or repairing, the total time must be allowed. If the staff are reassigned to other activities or use another piece of equipment, however, the time the equipment or room is down for service should not be counted.

Meetings other than inservice or education

It seems as though organizations cannot exist without meetings, and when there are changes occurring there are even more meetings. If volume is dropping, there are meetings to determine why, to determine how to prevent further drops, to decide how to generate new volume, and finally, to decide how to explain to the staff what management is doing. For many managers, meetings can consume the majority of each day. Routine meetings that should be identified and the time for them quantified include hospital department head and supervisory meetings, departmental meetings (typically monthly), sectional or shift meetings, and committee meetings. In nursing and in some other departments, there is also the routine change of shift meeting.

It is necessary to quantify the number of staff attending the meetings, as well as meeting frequency, duration, and preparation, and the amount of follow-up time spent (e.g., pulling records or reports, preparing material for review, or preparing minutes). It may be possible to combine meetings to save time or to report to staff the results of meetings rather than having more staff actually attend every meeting.

It may be possible to combine meetings to save time or to report to staff the results of meetings rather than having more staff actually attend every meeting.

Orientation

It is necessary to identify and quantify the time for both new employee orientation and for orientation of existing employees to new equipment or procedures. For example, hospitals or departments being computerized must allow time for staff to learn how to use the system.

New employee orientation is a function of the turnover rate rather than the size of the department. In stable departments, the turnover rate may be 10 percent or less. In other departments, particularly those with many part-time staff, the rate may be 40 percent or more. In support departments the orientation may be very structured and last one week or less. In professional or technical departments it may take several months of orientation to enable the employees to function independently. Functioning independently may mean the ability to take charge, work alternate shifts, work in several sections, or work on a wide variety of procedures. In practice, a new employee is of very limited, perhaps of zero value, and eventually is worth 100 percent. The learning process is called a *learning curve*. For administrative ease, management engineers typically count a new employee as zero value for some amount of time and as 100 percent thereafter. Thus, for example four weeks of orientation would be allowed for a new nurse or technologist.

Purchasing and supply activities

While purchasing and supply may be part of the already identified time of a supervisor or clerical person, if other personnel perform the function the time needs to be quantified. This includes interviewing vendors, at-tending demonstrations within the institution, preparing weekly orders, and receiving and putting supplies away on shelves or in storerooms. If this takes more than one percent of total staff time, it may be appropriate to investigate methods of reducing the time, by using, for example, standing orders, a central materiel management system, or a review of standard stock levels.

Quality control activities

Quality control occurs in many departments ranging from housekeeping to technical departments to nursing. If not quantified as part of management, it is necessary to measure the time spent. This may include use of computers or preparation of monthly reports. In some departments it may be a full-time staff assignment, while in others it may be part of the work of many individuals.

Research and development

Many consider research and development activities to be limited to a teaching hospital or specialty cost center. Development of a new test or procedures to bring tests in-house, evaluation of methods or equipment, procedure writing, etc., however, occur in most departments. Research and development could also include the time spent preparing a paper for publication.

Standby or idle time

While not an activity per se, idle time is a legitimate occurrence in many departments particularly on the evening or night shift. It could occur on any shift near the end of the employee tour when the work is completed (e.g., the operating rooms). In addition, the nature of certain departments, such as labor and delivery and the emergency department, requires some standby time. If idle time is too great a percentage (typically more than 5 percent to 10 percent) of total staff time, it may be necessary to make staffing adjustments. These could take the form of staggered shifts, elimination of an evening or night shift, or transfer of work from one department to another.

ANALYSIS METHODS

Nonwidget-producing activities may take less than 5 percent of the worked time in some departments but more commonly take between 15 percent and 25 percent of total worked time. A reduction in this time should result in a reduction in the cost of the service, provided that the reduction is real. If the activity is eliminated or the time spent is reduced but the result is an increase in standby or idle time, the staff may be happier, but there has been no savings.

There are three common methods for quantifying the time spent on nonwidget-producing activities. They are interviews, employee diaries, and direct observation. The decision on which method to use should be based on the size of the department staff and the degree of accuracy desired.

An interview can last more than one hour, and the accuracy of the information obtained varies based on the skills of the interviewer, the knowledge of the interviewee, and the ability of the interviewee to quantify time. If the department is open seven days per week or three shifts per day, it may be necessary to conduct several interviews in order to get an accurate picture of time spent on nonwidget-producing activities. Some staff may hesitate to say that there is standby or idle time for fear of losing their jobs or of having to work harder.

Employee diaries are a common method of collecting data from a large staff. The length of the data collection may be one week to one month depending on the variation in activities. Some activities may occur on a monthly cycle even though they take several hours or days to complete. A danger with using diaries is that some employees may expand the time spent on some activities to show that they were working the entire shift rather than showing standby time. This can be overcome by having the supervisors monitor the diary completion or by monitoring the process daily.

Direct observation is the most time-consuming approach and requires a trained observer. For activities that occur only a minor percentage of the time, it may be necessary to make several hundred observations in order to ensure that the time estimates are correct. Even a skilled observer may not know exactly what is happening. For instance, if a person is observed using the telephone, it is not known if the call was business related or personal.

It may be best to discuss the situation with the supervisors and staff. Explain why a study of nonwidget-producing activities is taking place and solicit their input as to how best to identify and quantify the time spent. They are also the persons who are most likely to know of ways to reduce or eliminate the unnecessary time.

•   •   •

No one works 100 percent of the time and any department with more than one employee is going to have some nonwidget-producing activities. Even the act of being paid requires someone to approve the timecard. These activities, including standby and idle time, are essential but have a cost associated with them.

Health care is competitive and will become more competitive. Managers must learn to work smarter rather than harder; they must continually review what is happening in their departments to remain productive and to become more productive. It is costly and dangerous to spend too much time on nonwidget-producing activities, but it is also short-sighted to spend too little time. In the short run one can reduce inservice or preventive maintenance and can avoid replacing and orienting new staff, but it all catches up in the long run.

Quality management demands an ongoing awareness of the components of work in every department. Sustained and improved productivity can occur only as a result of continuous hard work. Whatever widget a department produces, there is a faster, cheaper, or better way to produce it. The manager's job is to find that way and to implement it.

REFERENCES

1. Templin, J.L., Jr. "Productivity and the Supervisor." *The Health Care Supervisor* 1, no. 3 (1983):2.
2. Templin, J.L., Jr. "Productivity Monitoring for Every Supervisor." *The Health Care Supervisor* 2, no. 4 (1984):36–37.
3. Ibid.
4. Committee on Workload Recording. *Manual For Laboratory Workload Recording Method.* Skokie, Ill.: College of American Pathologists, 1986, p. 125.

Work simplification: a supervisor's challenge

Kenneth P. Cohen
President
Kalmain Management Systems
Woodland Hills, California

QUESTION: "Why do you do it this way?" Answer: Because that's the way we've always done it!" Have you, as a supervisor, ever asked the foregoing question of one of your employees or coworkers, an employee in another department, a vendor or your department head? And was the reply much the same? If so, did you: (1) accept the answer and go about your business; (2) ignore the answer and proceed to demonstrate a different technique; or (3) stop to analyze the situation and determine if an improved method could or should be developed?

Because a task has always been done the same way, does that make it right for today? Are buggy whips still made the way they were made at the turn of the century? Of course, this is a facetious question. Because of work simplification and advances in technology, we no longer *need* buggy

Health Care Superv, 1983,2(1),12–21

whips. In fact, a prime requisite of work simplification is determination of need.

WHY IMPROVE METHODS?

About 30 years ago, *Administrative Management* featured the following in bold letters on one of its monthly covers: "If something has been done the same way for 10 years, it can probably be improved by changing it." The editors of that journal were not advocating change for the sake of change. They recognized, however, that methods tend to stagnate over time and that we should constantly seek better ways of doing things. They were also acknowledging that environments, technology and management all change.

Who could have predicted just ten years ago that the personal computer would be as popular as it is today? What do the next five years hold in store for us in health care? Will advances that most of us cannot dream of today then be commonplace?

But *why* should better ways of doing things be sought? Do you, as a health care supervisor, feel that you perform all your functions in the most productive method possible? Is your staff performing its assigned tasks in the most cost-effective manner, or do you wish that you could accomplish your department's work with nine rather than ten persons? Do you sometimes feel that some of your employees could be more productive, but you feel unsure as to how to guide them to this end? Finally, are you sometimes frustrated in your attempts to solve certain departmental problems?

If any of the foregoing describes your situation, do not despair. A solution is available: *work simplification.* First, however, to determine the role of work simplification in the health care field and put it in the proper perspective, a few terms must be defined.

KEY CONCEPTS

Systems

Webster's Seventh New Collegiate Dictionary defines a system as "an organization forming a network for serving a common purpose." In a hospital, the network of functions that interrelate to serve the common purpose of patient care includes all services provided by the hospital (e.g., admitting, nursing, ancillary clinical services, medical records, dietary and social services).

Each function within the organization relates either directly or indirectly to the network of functions having the ultimate goal of seeing the patient through the various steps of the health care process. In effect, the hospital environment can be envisioned as comprising many systems and subsystems, each related, overlapping, dynamic and contributing to the improvement of patient care.

Methods improvement

Methods improvement is a general term that refers to making changes for the better in the means used to accomplish work. Such means include any or all of the managerial, supervisory and operational practices used in achieving desired results. It is the general philosophy of seeking to improve the way things are done.

Methods improvement applies to all activities, including improvements in such diverse areas as medical staff relations, fund raising, nursing activities, computer inputting and purchasing. Methods improvement activities range from informal, unorganized attempts to achieve a better way to the establishment of a formal program that is funded and supported by the organization. The latter is usually accomplished by establishing a formal management engineering department.

Work simplification

Work simplification refers to the systematic use of common sense in the quest for better and easier methods of accomplishing work.[1] Nadler says that work simplification is the systematic analysis of any type of work to: (1) eliminate unnecessary work, (2) arrange remaining work in the best order possible and (3) make certain that the right method is used.[2] Put more simply, it is organized common sense.

Common sense suggests an average degree of reliable ability to judge and decide with soundness, prudence and intelligence, without sophistication or special knowledge. Most people have (or believe they

have) common sense. *Organized* common sense takes that sound, prudent judgment and gives it direction and purpose. This is what we should hope to develop as health care supervisors.

Management engineers use sophisticated tools to perform their assignments: process charts, flow diagrams, operation charts, multiple activity charts, work sampling studies, micromotion studies, time studies, statistical studies, specialized computer programs, etc. However, the tools discussed herein are much more basic and can be applied by anyone without specialized engineering training. These tools are especially appropriate for supervisors who must accomplish the work of their departments through the efforts of other people.

THE MAKE-READY, DO AND PUT-AWAY PHENOMENON

Every task that can be performed by human beings consists of a "make-ready, do and put-away" sequence of activities. Consider, for example, a task that is performed often by homeowners—watering the lawn. Note the following sequence:

- *Make ready:* The homeowner walks to the garage where the hose reel is stored, rolls the reel to the front lawn hose bibb and connects the hose to the bibb.
- *Do:* The homeowner turns on the water and sprays a portion of the lawn for approximately 15 minutes while unreeling the hose from the reel as required.

- *Put away:* After a section of the lawn has been watered sufficiently, the homeowner turns off the water, disconnects the hose from the bibb and winds the hose onto the reel.

After the first section of lawn has been watered, the sequence is repeated section after section until the homeowner is satisfied that all areas of the lawn are adequately watered. Also, as part of the final put-away sequence, the homeowner rolls the hose reel back to the garage for storage. The description of the make-ready and put-away elements may differ slightly as each section of lawn is covered, but the concept of the three elements can readily be visualized.

As a health care supervisor, has your department head ever asked you to estimate how much time a certain task would take your group to accomplish? Did you make a time estimate based on all three elements: the make-ready, the do and the put-away? Or did you estimate the *do* portion only, without being fully aware of the other two elements? If so, do not worry; in such a case, it is usual to think only of the *productive* element and overlook the other two essentially *nonproductive* elements. And yet the make-ready and the put-away elements of a task are frequently more time consuming than the do element. However, it is important to realize that every task consists of all three elements.

A medical technologist performs a specific test by making ready (e.g., as-sembling reagents, test tubes and pipettes), doing the test (actually performing the test) and putting away (e.g., breaking down the setup, clearing away equipment and supplies and writing test results on the appropriate form). A business office clerk (collector) attempting to collect an overdue bill makes ready (selects the appropriate file and reviews the necessary information), does the task (makes a telephone call, discusses payment terms with the ex-patient and hangs up the phone) and puts away (makes notations in the file, sets up a reminder file for later follow-through and files the chart).

By visualizing every task in this manner, it is possible to become more productive in work simplification efforts. The objective is to reduce the *nonproductive* elements (make-ready and put-away) to bare minimum and to make the *productive element* (do) even more productive.

SCIENTIFIC APPROACH TO PROBLEM SOLVING

Most health care supervisors have been exposed to the scientific approach to problem solving, probably in relation to solving problems in their own technical fields. The same general approach can be applied to supervisory problems. About 25 years ago, in a supervisory training class held at a large midwestern hospital, the hospital's executive director asked, "Why are we concentrating on problem solving? We want to teach our department heads and supervisors how to *manage.*" The instructor's reply was, "What is management but the ability to recognize and solve *problems?*" The executive director asked no more questions.

In their problem-solving approaches, authorities enumerate varying numbers of steps, usually ranging from 5 to 12. The number of steps is unimportant; what is important, however, is the sequence and the logic to be followed. A recommended approach uses the following eight steps:

1. Define the problem.
2. Collect relevant data.
3. Analyze the data.
4. Develop alternative solutions.
5. Select the best solution.
6. Implement the selected solution.
7. Follow up on results.
8. Refine the system.

Define the problem

Defining the problem is by far the most critical and important step in problem solving. An ancient seer once said, "A problem well stated is half solved." To write out a problem definition clearly and succinctly, framing it in the best possible language so that all concerned with the problem understand and agree that the written statement fairly defines the problem, is often a difficult task. However, care taken at this step will reduce the time, effort, resources and ultimate cost of a project.

Our usual tendency is to state, "Here is my problem." Almost imme-

Care taken in defining the problem will reduce the time, effort, resources and ultimate cost of a project.

diately we then add, "And here is my solution to that problem." Many persons attempt this shortcut approach to problem solving. However, such shortcuts are costly in human effort and physical resources. It is essential to follow the sequence described here for the best and least costly results.

Collect relevant data

When collecting data, the management engineer determines which tools appear best suited for collecting data related to the stated problem. However, the technical tools used by the management engineer are unnecessary for the health care supervisor. Work simplification deals with organized common sense, and experience has shown repeatedly that the best tools for this purpose are paper, pencil and an inquiring mind.

In the lawn-watering situation mentioned earlier, assume that a homeowner spends two hours daily on this task. Assume further that the problem definition from step 1 is:

Determine a method of watering 2,000 square feet of lawn daily in the summer so that each square foot of lawn is watered for approximately 15 minutes, so that the homeowner's time spent on this task will consume 20 minutes or less each day.

Using action verbs, short narrative descriptions of each step in the task should be written. Since considerable walking is involved in the task, a column entitled *distance* could be inserted for the number of feet walked for each appropriate step. The goal is to reduce the amount of time spent by the homeowner, so distance walked might be significant. (A comfortable walking rate is approximately 200 feet per minute.) Another column for approximate time could be included for those steps that do not require walking.

The data collection sheet should be as detailed and specific as possible. The more detailed the data, the easier the subsequent analysis. A partial sample of a data collection sheet, using the lawn-watering example, is shown in Figure 1.

Analyze the data

When analyzing the data, six questions should be asked about each step of the task: who? what? where? when? how? and why? They can be asked in any sequence as long as each question is asked at each step in the task shown on the data collection sheet. The most important of these questions is always *why?*

Who performs this step, and *why* does he or she perform it? Could it be performed better by someone with less skill? Is the person with the necessary skills performing this step? *Why* must this step be performed at

Present Method

Description	Approximate time (min.)	Distance (ft.)
1. Walk from kitchen to hose reel in garage		35
2. Wheel hose reel to front lawn (section 1)		70
3. Unroll hose and position nozzle end		25
4. Walk length of hose and fit hose end to bibb		25
5. Turn on water		
6. Walk length of hose and pick up nozzle		25
7. Spray water in arc	15	
8. Place nozzle on ground and walk hose length		25
9. Turn off water		
10. Wind hose onto reel	3	
11. Wheel reel to front lawn (section 2)		110
. . . etc.	. . .	. . .
Total*	108	2800
Equivalent @ 200 ft./min.	14	
Total	122	

* Included in the approximate time total are figures from the additional steps required that are not listed in this figure.

Figure 1. Sample data collection sheet.

all? If the step must be performed, what skills must be used?

What is being done in this step? Why must it be performed at all? Can it be eliminated? If not, can it be shortened, lengthened, reduced, expanded, etc.? In short, question every conceivable aspect of what is being done, and why it is being done, for each step.

Where is this task being performed? Why must it be performed in the laboratory (or wherever it is now being performed)? Maybe it would better be performed in. . . .

When is the step performed? Why must it be performed at a certain time of day, a particular day of the week, a specific day of the month, etc.? When would this step be performed better? What happens when this step is now performed at . . . ? What would happen if this step were to be performed at . . . ?

How is this task being performed now? Why must it be performed in this manner? What would happen if this step were performed in another manner? If the sequence of steps were to change, how would this affect the final result? If one or two or more steps were to be eliminated, how would it affect the final outcome? Was the sequence ever changed before? If so, what was changed? How was the task performed previously? Can something new be learned by delving into past practices?

Finally, ask again the *why* question. Why is this operation being performed at all? If it must be performed, why does a nurse (or clerk,

technologist, secretary, dietitian, etc.) perform this step? Why is this step performed at this particular place? Why at this particular time? Why in this particular manner? Why in this particular sequence?

In using the questioning approach for analyzing the present lawn-watering method, the homeowner would have to ask the following and other questions. Why must one walk more than one-half mile each time the lawn is watered? How can the lawn be adequately watered while reducing the amount of walking? Why must one spend two hours daily in this activity? Since considerable physical effort must be expended in the present method, how can the number of sequential steps be reduced? Can the lawn be watered in fewer than six sections? Would the purchase of a 75-foot hose to replace the 50-foot hose in use reduce the number of sections? Would a sprinkler system be practical? What would it cost? Would automatic timers help to reduce the time taken? What would they cost?

Develop alternative solutions

After asking the questions exhaustively for each step shown on the data collection sheet, various alternatives to the present method should begin to present themselves. Each logical sequence of steps must then be documented similarly to the present method. Label options as proposed method A, proposed method B, etc.

In the lawn-watering example, assume that the homeowner develops three solutions. Method A involves a method similar to the present method except that a new 75-foot-long hose is purchased, so that the lawn need only be divided into three sections. This reduces the total watering time for the homeowner to 40 minutes with an expenditure of $60.

Method B involves installing lawn sprinklers throughout the property, thus eliminating the handling of the hose and hose reel, and connecting and disconnecting from the hose bibbs. The homeowner does considerably less walking because the method requires only the manual turning on and off of the water valves that control six sections of lawn.

The total time for the homeowner to walk to the valves, turn them on and off and return to the house is 18 minutes per day. However, the homeowner must be in or near the house for the full two-hour span that is required to water all six sections sequentially (the control function). The capital investment is $600.

Method C is similar to Method B except that automatic timers are added as control devices to eliminate the necessity for manually controlling the water valves. This reduces the time spent by the homeowner to almost nothing. The capital expenditure over the present method is $750.

Select the best solution

After all solutions have been documented, analyze each solution in relation to the problem definition. At a minimum, four factors must be evaluated to permit selection of the most feasible solution. No single factor is the most important; the factors vary in importance in relation to the work being studied. The factors are:

- economic;
- hazard;
- control; and
- psychological.

Wherever possible, a dollar amount should be affixed to each step in the process. If the new steps save dollars, such savings should be shown as pluses on the proposed methods worksheet. If the new steps will cost dollars to implement, such as the purchase of supplies and equipment or additional labor, these costs should be shown as minuses. The algebraic sum of the pluses and minuses will represent the net savings of the proposed method.

A proposed methods summary for the lawn-watering example is shown in Figure 2. Method A requires the smallest investment, but it involves more physical hazards than the other two methods. And because it ties up the homeowner for 40 minutes daily, it presents the worst psychological disadvantage. Method B requires ten times the investment of Method A, but it presents fewer physical hazards, offers better control and is better psychologically for the homeowner. Method C requires 25 percent more investment than Method B (1,150 percent greater investment than Method A), but it is obviously the best choice from the hazard, control and psychological standpoints.

At this point, the homeowner must

Proposed methods	Factors			
	Economic	Hazard	Control	Psychological
A	$60 investment	Physical handling, possible tripping	Easy	Worst
B	$600 investment	Much less	Better	Better
C	$750 investment	Nil	Best	Best

Figure 2. Sample proposed methods worksheet.

make a management decision. All four factors must be weighed carefully to determine if the conditions detailed in step 1, problem definition, have been satisfied by each of the proposed methods. Analysis of all factors in Method A shows that the time factor was reduced from 2 hours to 40 minutes, but this exceeds the 20-minute criterion defined in step 1. Method A would be eliminated, leaving only Methods B and C. Comparing Methods B and C the homeowner must decide if the extra $150 investment for Method C would be worth the reduction in time, the virtual elimination of physical hazards and the improved control over the process.

Implement, follow-up and refine

To implement the results of step 5, certain mechanical or physical changes must be made. Personnel may have to be trained. Procedures may have to be documented. Other departments' activities may have to be modified, expanded, contracted or otherwise altered. If such is the case, other department heads must be brought into the cycle at a very early stage.

Once changes have been made, procedures have been documented and personnel have been trained, the new method should be tested and refined before final implementation.

The new method should be monitored closely to make certain that all elements work together as designed.

The new method should be monitored closely for a time to make certain that all elements work together as designed.

At this stage, the department head or supervisor must review the written procedures to ascertain that the documented procedures are being carried out properly by the personnel assigned to the new or revised tasks. Forms, equipment, supplies, etc., must be checked to make certain they function as planned. Controls developed during the prior steps must be verified to ensure that they are functioning properly and are actually *con-*

trolling the achievement of the desired results.

During the follow-up (step 7), possible refinements to the system may present themselves to the supervisor. Such refinements may suggest that a different solution (step 4) may be better in practice than the one selected. If so, steps 4 through 8 should again be followed after the new "best" solution has been developed.

In refining the system it may become apparent that the problem definition was not fully or accurately stated. In such a case, it may be necessary to rework the problem definition (step 1) and proceed again through all eight steps.

The scientific approach to problem solving is not cast in stone. Rather, it can be altered and adapted as conditions dictate. It is dynamic rather than static. Although it is a powerful tool, it is not an exact science. Above all, it is an iterative process, as illustrated in Figure 3.

As one completes the first seven steps, refinements will suggest themselves and may result in reentering the cycle at any one of the earlier steps and continuing through again to step 8. Since the process is iterative, the flow may be repeated until the designer (department head or supervisor) is satisfied that the method has been improved.

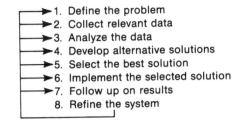

Figure 3. The process of problem solving in the scientific approach.

BASIC TOOLS

The challenge is clear: The supervisor's overall responsibility includes work simplification. The principles of analysis involved can be applied to everyday work activities. Nothing other than common sense is needed. No special training or technology is required; the only supplies needed are paper and pencil. But paramount and implicit in the process of work simplification is an inquiring mind.

The make-ready, do and put-away phenomenon is applicable to every human task, and the tools of utmost importance in the iterative problem-solving approach are the six questions: who? what? where? when? how? and why? Use your organized common sense to make improvements within that part of the health care organization for which you are responsible.

REFERENCES

1. Smalley, H.E. *Hospital Management Engineering.* Englewood Cliffs, N.J.: Prentice-Hall, 1982, p. 20.

2. Nadler, G. *Work Simplification.* New York: McGraw-Hill, 1957, p. 2.

Part III
Involvement for Improvement

Human resources management: keystone for productivity

Bruce M. Bartels
Vice President for Operations
Medical Center Hospital of
*   Vermont*

Keith L. Gee
Employee Relations Specialist
Medical Center Hospital of
*   Vermont*
Burlington, Vermont

T HE RELATIONSHIP between institutional productivity efforts and employee behavior often takes a back seat in the development of productivity improvement programs. A more common action is to use traditional management engineering techniques as the sole or primary approach. This article will explore the thinking behind a multifaceted productivity improvement effort that encompasses the quantitative disciplines required in any such undertaking and the less tangible human components.

Many improvement efforts, while initially successful, fail to bring about lasting productivity or quality improvements.[1] There have been costly negative results in some cases, including deterioration of quality and productivity as well as heightened labor strife.

A critical determinant of the success or failure of an effort to improve

Health Care Superv, 1987, 5(2), 47–53
© 1987 Aspen Publishers, Inc.

productivity is the breadth of purpose that management communicates for the effort.[2] The more successful organizations view their primary objectives as building a competitive, productive organization.[3] The unsuccessful organization focuses more narrowly on fine tuning existing activities, often at the cost of overlooking opportunities to correct inherent weaknesses and limitations in mission, product lines, strategies, cultures, structures, human resources, and technologies.

The question thus presented is: How do we include the concepts necessary to addressing lasting improvement in a productivity enhancement effort? Research would indicate that to successfully cope with increasingly hostile environments organizations should adopt a total systems improvement approach.[4] There are five key tasks that need to be accomplished in order to build the understanding, commitment, capabilities, and methodology necessary for improvement activities to succeed. These tasks are:

1. developing a common perspective on productivity;
2. developing a culture supportive of productivity improvement efforts;
3. maximizing human resources;
4. developing organization capabilities; and
5. continually searching for improvement.

While the foregoing tasks are listed serially, only the initial task need take place in the designated order.

Once a common perspective is achieved, the remaining items can be undertaken concurrently; they are in fact never fully completed, as they are ongoing activities in a thriving organization. The remainder of this article will examine these tasks and suggest a framework for productivity enhancement based upon them.

DEVELOPING A COMMON PERSPECTIVE ON PRODUCTIVITY

There are many different interpretations of the meaning and utilization of productivity. The varying perspectives that individuals have of productivity and the implications that they see may handicap an effort at enhancement. Clarity and consensus regarding terminology, purpose, and methodology need to be achieved.

An important element in developing a common perspective beyond that of mere definition is exposure to the reasoning behind the renewed emphasis on productivity. Among the forces now so familiar to us are:

- pressures from payers and consumers to provide the same or better quality service at equal or lower cost;
- prospective payment;
- market and price competition;
- availability of capital financing; and
- inflationary pressure on wages, benefits, supplies, utilities, and equipment.

A major factor in dealing with each of the foregoing issues is productivity improvement. Communication to hospital staff members of the positive, progressive elements of productivity improvement is critical. Leaving the impression that productivity is synonymous with austerity, loss of job security, sacrifices, or lower quality is unlikely to result in enthusiasm.

DEVELOPING A CULTURE SUPPORTIVE OF PRODUCTIVITY IMPROVEMENT

Much is being written these days about organizational culture.[5] It appears to be an essential ingredient for long-term success and is often the distinguishing characteristic between success and failure. A culture is a shared set of beliefs and behaviors. How can management set out to define and make productivity improvement a part of its culture and convince others to share in this undertaking?

There are three major steps in building a culture supportive of productivity improvement. The initial action is to define when necessary and communicate the institutional mission, values, and objectives, and to explain the role of productivity improvement in the accomplishment of these. The intent is to develop a sense of purpose behind the productivity improvement effort. Many repeated acts achieve this. Among them are periodic presentation and discussion of corporate productivity objectives in settings available to all employees; articles in internal pub-

lications; incorporation of these concepts in the annual planning cycle; and identification of this notion in performance evaluations. The awareness that is created by these actions must then be translated into commitment. Commitment is the most elusive step in developing this facet of a culture, but once it occurs individuals can collectively pursue the objective.

There are no certain ways to achieve commitment. However, commitment should spring from a common perspective of individual and organizational well-being. When there is a high degree of congruence with regard to the presence and form of threats and opportunities it is most likely that commitment will be achieved.

One mechanism for communicating that productivity improvement is a standard expectation of every staff member's job is its incorporation as an element of job performance.

One mechanism for communicating that productivity improvement is a standard expectation of every staff member's job is its incorporation as an element of job performance. A vehicle that serves this purpose is a process called performance contracting.[6]

Performance contracting is a modification of management by objectives

(MBO). It uses as a communication vehicle a set of mutually agreed upon objectives directed toward obtaining results in specific areas. The performance agreement has an impact far beyond its use as an evaluation or appraisal tool. The key areas identified for results are those that senior management selects as critical to the organization's interests for the coming year. This process has a cascading communications impact. As senior management selects key result areas, divisional and departmental managers identify objectives that represent the desired results. Discussion and negotiation between managers, which must occur to complete a performance contract, reinforce institutional direction and priority.

The requirement for identification of individual actions supporting the direction established in performance contracting also permits "buying in" to occur. A manager takes an active role in creating and defining the tasks that will constitute achievement. A sensitivity to individual autonomy and participation is thus expressed through the contract.

Once a theme is developed and shared it may be made part of the organization's culture, but it must be sustained through recycling and reinforcement. This can be done by encouraging each department to define standards for productivity, promote employee involvement in improvement opportunities, increase employee recognition for achievement, and integrate standards of productivity in individual appraisals.

MAXIMIZING HUMAN RESOURCES

Attaining improvements in productivity and quality hinges on human behavior. Recognizing that each member of a hospital staff represents a potential to be tapped is central to identifying opportunities for improvement. There are several components to addressing the human aspect of this process. One is to develop and support a positive employee relations climate. Many interrelated actions are required to build these positive relations, and they all require attention to communication.

An organization's management should express its commitment to optimizing human resources in its corporate objectives and priorities. Management evaluation schemes should focus on employee relations. Additionally, policies, procedures, and practices should be reviewed with consideration for the extent to which they support a positive climate.

As basic as the foregoing is the requirement to provide managers and supervisors with tools to assist them in establishing, monitoring, and assessing a positive climate. Instruction in the creation of this environment should be undertaken. A human resources department should have the capacity to develop educational programs providing managers with training, consulting, and coaching on employee relations matters. Incentives to emphasize a positive climate can be built into performance evaluations.

Issues of job security will inevitably arise as change is suggested and greater productivity is pursued.[7] Addressing these concerns as an initial element of the process can be of benefit to the organization as well as to the individual. An employee who perceives his or her job as secure is more likely to be productive and less likely to seek security through other employment. Issues that might result from stress, such as health or family problems, may also be minimized.

Job security, it should be noted, is not intended to mean an absolute guarantee of employment. It does, however, mean that the employer must be concerned about the welfare of the employees and must strive to project that concern. Once again, communication is key. A clear understanding of the employer's long-range plans regarding labor planning and an explanation of the environment generating these plans should be conveyed to all employees.

The organization's policies and practices dealing with work force reductions should be sensitive to employee concerns and should be known and available to all. When specific actions causing change occur, explanations of such events should be provided through in-house publications and other appropriate media. Such action will decrease the extent of incorrect information that is spread by word of mouth.

As higher levels of performance are sought through enhancements in productivity, recognition and reward for performance should become part of an organization's culture.[8] Financial and other incentives for improvement, recognition through an award system, and performance-based pay systems each have a place in developing the shared value of greater productivity. It goes almost without saying that promotion of the involvement of individual employees is a significant requirement in seeking to improve an organization's productivity.

The following should be considered when determining how to promote involvement:

- explanatory seminars on approaches used in other organizations;
- a forum giving individual managers the opportunity to demonstrate methods they have used effectively;
- training sessions in problem-solving skills for employee groups; and
- the requirement that each department select an involvement approach appropriate to its unique needs.

DEVELOPING ORGANIZATIONAL CAPABILITIES

A number of supportive capabilities must be present to sustain an ongoing productivity improvement effort. The first such required capability is the expertise to establish a productivity measurement system.[9] If productivity is to be objectively evaluated and improved, indicators for each area of activity need to be developed. This information is required to meet a number of needs. Indicators that are simple, easy to explain, and quickly calculated will help in monitoring and controlling performance. Comparative indicators that measure how an area compares with industrywide standards provide useful information as well as a competitive objective. As these indicators are developed, a method for producing relevant management reports on a periodic basis should be established as well.

As productivity can be a complex topic involving many disciplines, establishing a technical support group should be considered.

As productivity can be a complex topic involving many disciplines, establishing a technical support group should be considered.[10] This group would be available to guide and consult on various efforts taking place throughout the organization.

Representatives from several areas should be involved in the technical support group—at least membership from management engineering, quality control, personnel, data processing, and finance. Such a group can identify and catalogue institutionwide activity, provide information and expertise not generally available, and develop consistency and continuity for diverse endeavors.

Assessment tools may be as valuable as any single aid in determining where to begin.[11] Everyone becomes conditioned to their environment over time, and opportunities for change may become less visible. Assessment tools provide a structured approach to review existing systems, policies, practices, and procedures. Such tools include:

- employee relations reports;
- opinion surveys;
- internal audits;
- work simplification, work sampling, and downtime studies;
- work flow and space–relationship analyses; and
- purchasing audits and studies.

Another essential support activity is the development of a resource library.[12] This collection may be overseen by the technical support group. It should serve as a repository for information from all disciplines bearing on the topic of productivity. An organized approach for making this information available should be developed for the purpose of keeping abreast of recent developments as well as maintaining productivity efforts in a highly visible fashion.

THE ONGOING SEARCH FOR IMPROVEMENT

The final task is to continue pursuing the creation of a corporate culture having productivity as one of its primary values. Underlying this value is the assumption that anything and everything—product, cost, process, attitude, and interactions—can be improved. The integration of productivity and quality to produce greater value should be viewed as an overriding objective. It is this result that generates the rewards for initially undertaking productivity enhancement efforts.

Improvement efforts are aimed at all levels of the organization. The individual employee must be brought into the process. This may occur through various management strategies such as pay for performance, management by objectives, or quality circles. Individual actions and ideas need to be harnessed to work group, departmental, or divisional objectives. This permits capture and transmission of important innovations that benefit the activities of the group.

Integrating and supporting functions should occur at the corporate level so that achievement is recognized and enlarged upon. Supporting resources can be used to augment individual or small-group efforts and may be most effectively provided by a staff available to many people.

The new organizational culture is generated by a multidisciplinary approach aimed at various levels of the organization and arrayed in such a way as to develop a cyclic and reinforcing process. The support of individual and group efforts in pursuit of productivity that addresses the needs and experiences of the people involved will create the highest probability of success. The recognition and support of the human resources that drive productivity serve the best interests of any organization; only through behavioral change will lasting improvement be achieved.

REFERENCES

1. Goodman, P.S. "Why Productivity Programs Fail: Reasons and Solutions." *National Productivity Review* 1 (Autumn 1982): 369–80.
2. Metz, E.J. "Managing Change: Implementing Productivity and Quality Improvements." *National Productivity Review* 3 (Summer 1984) 303–13.
3. Moss, S. "A Systems Approach to Productivity." *National Productivity Review* 3 (Summer 1984) 270–79.
4. Ibid., 271.
5. Deal, T.E., and Kennedy, A.A. *Corporate Cultures.* Reading, Mass.: Addison-Wesley, 1982.
6. McDonald, C.R. *MBO Can Work! How to Manage By Contract.* New York: McGraw–Hill, 1982.
7. Mooney, M. "Organizing for Productivity Management." *National Productivity Review* 1 (Spring 1982): 141–50.
8. Shetty, Y.K. "Key Elements of Productivity Improvement Programs." *Business Horizons* 25 (March–April 1982): 15–22.
9. Kendrick, J.W. *Improving Company Productivity.* Baltimore, Md.: Johns Hopkins University Press, 1984, p. 118.
10. Bureau of Business Practice. "Centering the Productivity/Quality Effort." *Productivity Improvement Bulletin*, no. 407, January 10, 1984, 1–3.
11. Mooney, "Organizing for Productivity Management," 148.
12. Ibid., 146.

The importance of
Japanese management
to health care supervisors:
Quality and American circles

Robert Boissoneau
Special Adviser to the President
Visiting Professor
Wright State University
Dayton, Ohio

A SUBJECT frequently discussed today is Japanese management. In America this topic usually arises when addressing issues surrounding employee involvement in the work setting.

In the process of helping to rebuild Japan after World War II, the progressive ideas of American social scientists, behaviorists, and engineers such as W. Edwards Deming and Joseph M. Juran were introduced to Japanese managers. With the assistance of these Americans, Japanese managers applied employee participation measures in their organizations. This reapplication of American thinking to American organizational relationships after the success in Ja-

Barbara Sagarin, former director of the Productivity Group in Tempe, Arizona, contributed many of the ideas stated in this article.

Robert Boissoneau is on sabbatical leave from Arizona State University, Tempe.

Health Care Superv, 1987, 5(3), 28–38
© 1987 Aspen Publishers, Inc.

pan has been referred to as Theory Z. The American principles, essentially focusing on the worth of workers, have been used by the Japanese to improve national productivity.

Recent American critics of Japanese management applications in this country point out the vast differences between the two cultures and, consequently, between the two sets of workers. They quickly state that Theory Z will not be effective in this country.

Reflective supporters of the Japanese method are not declaring that a verbatim translation of management–labor relationships from Japan to the United States should occur. They are saying, however, that American managers should at least review the practices of Japanese management; most observers feel that the Japanese appear to have had great success. Thus, American managers should apply in their own firms those practices that they believe are applicable in this country.

Most people agree that not everything would work in the United States. For example, it is difficult to imagine American workers going to work early for calisthenics on the organization's lawn. Certainly, differences between the two cultures do exist.

CULTURAL DIFFERENCES

In Japan, management is more paternalistic than it is in America. Managers in Japan are interested in the lives of workers beyond the work place. They feel a loyalty toward each worker, so much so that if a worker is not performing effectively the poor performance is taken to indicate the manager's lack of interest.

American management is more autocratic than paternalistic, but it is still more paternalistic than democratic. The workers' obligation to the company in the United States is confined to the normal workday. After-hours connections are usually limited to such activities as bowling leagues and softball games, and little loyalty is displayed by American managers toward workers. In addition, more often than in the United States, Japanese workers remain with the same firm for an entire career.

Working men and women in this country often maintain an adversarial relationship with management. This is in part due to the history of autocratic management in this society, but it also exists because of the aggressiveness of people in our culture. In contrast, the Japanese personality is less assertive.

Managers and workers in Japan take a cooperative approach to decision making. A participative decision-making approach is used by management to form an arrangement in which employee involvement is solicited. The effect of such a decision-making process is that the planning or collection-of-data phase in Japan is longer than that found in U.S. management. However, as Japanese management spends time talking with workers about various issues that affect workers, it is building rapport and credibility that enables the implementation phase following the decision to be shortened.

By contrast, in America management does not spend much time talking with workers in the data-collection phase of the typical decision, but rather spends much more time with implementation than its Japanese counterpart. After a decision has been made and implemented, American managers typically spend time selling the decision to others, including employees.

Regarding management control of workers, U.S. managers must be more explicit than Japanese managers. Where administrators of American institutions go to great lengths to be precise and definite in establishing controls and related communication, Japanese managers can be much less specific in the direction they provide. Japanese managers trust their workers more than American managers do. The relationship between workers and management in Japan assumes many of the characteristics of a family; few organizations in the United States follow this pattern.

Japanese organizational behavior philosophy states that both workers and management are responsible for ensuring the firm's effectiveness. The total effort of all people concerned is important in Japan, and group effort is supreme. In Japan, individuals are not singled out for either praise or scorn.

In comparison, America is a much more individualistic society. Organizations honor individual attainment in our culture. Various types of recognition, such as Employee of the Month and other personnel devices, are widely used to honor outstanding individual workers. Through the practice of individual performance appraisal, managers are able to identify not only positive performance but negative features as well. Appraising the individual is important in all phases of life, including school and sports. This is part of our cultural heritage.

At work, employees of Japanese companies expect that pay increases and job promotions will accrue slowly. In the current group environment in Japan, sharing information is widespread. An open climate characterizes the relationship between workers and management. All for one and one for all is the motto. Long-term effectiveness is important to the Japanese, and this accounts for the slow and deliberate progression of pay and promotion. Short-range benefits are less important than in this country.

By comparison, U.S. employees are on a fast track. They expect pay increases and promotions quickly. Many American workers see themselves heading for the top of their fields, and they want immediate recognition. Thus, in this kind of environment short-range objectives take priority over long-range considerations.

Japanese workers are trained as generalists. Throughout their careers, the Japanese move from one position to another and from one department to another, usually remaining in the same company. By this method, Japanese firms are assured broad understanding by employees of the total organization. Therefore, employees, instead of supervisors and managers, can perform much of the coordination function themselves because they know so much about the company's overall goals.

Specialization is used more widely in the United States. The argument in its favor is that greater expertise and effectiveness result from specialization. The difference is that American workers know much about a limited range of activities while the Japanese know less about a broader range of activities. The coordination function, relating one program or department to others, is assumed automatically by supervisors and managers in the American society.

Health care organizations are highly specialized along departmental lines. Some of the employees are overly specialized and do not know a great deal about related departments. Consequently, department heads and administrators spend an inordinate amount of time on coordination to help the institution function as a unified whole.

Some, although not all, Japanese workers have been given a guarantee of lifetime employment. Primarily, the largest firms offer this benefit. In ensuring lifetime employment, Japanese companies once again give evidence of long-term interest both in the firm and in the employee. Funding of training programs takes a high

priority in management–employee relations. The payment of bonuses and profit sharing are used as motivational tools by many Japanese firms. The companies hire college graduates once a year and follow the practice of promoting employees from within the organization. Tradition and heritage are more important in Japan than in the United States; thus, the largest firms take the best graduates from the best universities as a status symbol, while less renowned firms take their employees on a descending-order basis.

Finally, Japanese managers take a holistic approach toward their personnel. They integrate the economic and social aspects of life for willing employees. No such concern is acceptable in America where people make a clear distinction between work life and home life. Freedom, independence, and individualism remain principles that Americans hold dear.

QUALITY CIRCLES

The single greatest contribution that the Japanese approach to management has made to the American organization is quality circles. A quality circle is a group of volunteer member-employees who meet every week or two for the purpose of maintaining and improving the quality of the organization's output. Quality circles are used widely in Japan and are increasingly being used in the United States. Many *Fortune 500* firms, including Lockheed and Honeywell, are using quality circles. However, only a small number of health care organizations have developed quality circles to any extent.

A quality circle is a continuing work group that consists of about 6 to 10 people. Meetings are structured by members themselves and focus only on problems that are directly related to members' work; a meeting is never a complaint session against management.

Quality circles offer several benefits to the organization and to individual employees. For the organization, the quality circle improves the quality of products or services by enabling employees who work directly with the output to state their observations and recommend changes in an organized way. Workers can be involved in making decisions that affect the future of the service or product.

The quality circle improves the quality of products and services by enabling employees to state their observations and recommend changes in an organized way.

In most firms, the suggestion box is the only method that personnel have in addition to face-to-face discussions with supervisors to influence the company's direction.

Quality circles enable people at the absolute lowest levels of the organization to influence decisions. These are the people who know the product or service best and can, unlike some managers, observe the impact of the service firsthand. Allowing as much decision making as possible at the lowest level in the organization has long been advocated by supporters of decentralized management.

Employees who have never taken the opportunity to communicate with others in either a lateral or hierarchical direction can do so through quality circles. Lateral communication with workers in other departments and programs is particularly vital.

By using quality circles, the organization gains from better management–labor relations. Perhaps for the first time workers can see, hear, and understand that management wants to produce a good product or service and treat employees fairly.

Viewing the organization in such a positive light motivates personnel to perform at high levels of effectiveness. Reduced absenteeism, tardiness, and employee pilferage should result.

Finally, in reviewing the advantages of quality circles for the organization, observation of the operation of the quality circle groups over time enables management to identify workers who have the potential to help the organization and themselves as managers.

In addition to improving the firm's performance, quality circles offer several advantages to an institution's employees. At quality circle meetings workers can voice their personal, work-related opinions. Thus, quality circles help increase the employees' feelings of self-worth and self-fulfillment.

Sometimes the quality circle is the first chance workers have to correct work-related problems that have been hampering them for a long time.

For certain individuals experiencing an extended need for socialization, the group dynamics aspects of quality circles offer a boost in morale. Usually American workers do not become involved in group decision making. When they do, some like it and others do not. The ones who do like group decision making usually find considerable satisfaction in their quality circle groups.

Quality circles enable employees to improve themselves by engaging in personal development. They read and become involved in discussions that may increase their value to the current employer or to other employers.

As with other human endeavors, quality circles have weaknesses as well as strengths. First, they can be costly. Time away from the job for the meeting and preparation time needed for the quality circle leaders, the company's quality circle facilitator, the steering committee, and top management add up to a substantial amount of institutional resources devoted to the program.

A cost-related problem not yet solved in most organizations employing quality circles is a plan for sharing the results of expense-reducing ideas with employees who recommend them. Personnel expect to share in any financial gain that the organization accrues as a result of quality circle work. To date, truly helpful guidelines are lacking.

Another problem with quality circles is the amount of time necessary to devote to them. They are time consuming for all people involved. They require time for both oral and written communications, and gathering statistical data may be time consuming, especially if new programs must be written.

Finally, some people feel that quality circles reduce productivity. This may be the harshest of all criticisms, because the quality circle movement is considered to be a major reason for the high productivity levels reached by the Japanese. The critics claim that the amount of time required for meetings and preparation by all the people involved takes too much time away from actual work. In their view, the amount of investment is not justified by the outcome.

Whether quality circles will ever make a significant impact in this country remains unclear. Many of the companies that are now using them successfully are the nation's most progressive organizations—*Theory Z* organizations. These firms already know the important role that the ordinary worker can play. In a sense, quality circles represent a technique that these companies can use to their advantage.

Concern needs to be raised about the thousands of organizations that have reviewed and rejected quality circles and about those organizations that have never looked seriously at quality circles at all. Are these reactionary and backward organizations? No clear answer exists. One fact is certain, however; an organization that places no value on its employees' input for improving the organization's performance will be opposed to quality circles.

AMERICAN CIRCLES

Barbara Sagarin, former Director of the Productivity Group in Tempe, Arizona, is credited with tracing the evolution of training aspects of quality and American circles. American circles were developed in response to the unique American culture reflecting differences among people and organizations. Japanese engineers identified quality control circles in 1962 to monitor the production of industrial workers through the use of various techniques such as check sheets, sampling, and cause-and-effect diagrams. As the movement progressed, it became known as quality circles in 1974 with the extension of the concept to include behavioral applications along with the earlier identified engineering methods. For the first time in quality circle applications, principles of group dynamics, listening, and organizational development became more widely used in public service organizations as well as in private firms. In 1982, the Productivity Group began to use the term *American Circles* to acknowledge the Americanization of the concept. The following lists advantages of American circles for the organization and employees:

Organizational advantages
- improves labor–management relations;
- improves quality;
- cuts raw material costs;
- improves attrition rate and cuts absenteeism;
- promotes job involvement;
- establishes an in-house pool of potential managers;
- encourages employees' motivation;
- allows managers to manage, not to do workers' jobs;
- permits decision making at the lowest logical level;
- opens new channels of communication both horizontally and vertically;
- involves employees in problem solving instead of problem identification; and
- improves attitudes.

Employee advantages
- puts them in charge of their jobs;
- promotes team building and identification;
- allows for personal rewards with group responsibility;
- establishes channels for workers to satisfy needs for socialization, ego satisfaction, and self-actualization;
- satisfies employees' needs for a self-improvement program;
- allows for professional growth of circle members and leaders;
- allows employees to be heard;
- promotes organizational pride and loyalty; and
- allows employees to solve the daily work-related problems that frustrate them.

Many health care organizations state that they have quality circle programs when in fact they do not.

In summary, many health care organizations state that they have quality circle programs when in fact they do not. They often have some form of group activity, but they do not have programs that meet the following characteristics of a true quality circle program:

- meets each week or at least every other week;
- is prearranged to last at least from one half to one-and-one-half hours;
- has members who are trained in check sheets, techniques of cooperative behavior, cause and effect diagrams, Pareto diagrams, brainstorming, small group communications, measurement techniques, and management presentations;
- is organized so that the leader, in conjunction with the facilitator, trains all members either during the first 8 to 12 meetings or by setting aside part of each meeting for training purposes (occasionally a combination of both approaches is used);
- has a leader who ensures that the meeting adheres to the agenda and that all members are encouraged to participate;
- does not permit any one person within the group to be made a scapegoat;

- addresses only those problems directly related to the work of the members (personalities and corporate policy do not fall under their jurisdiction);
- has a steering committee that meets regularly and takes an active role in ensuring that the environment is conducive to quality circles;
- has the continuing support of executive management; and
- uses cooperation as a tool to accomplish its goals.

IMPLICATIONS FOR HEALTH CARE SUPERVISORS

While there is little doubt that Japanese management and quality circles have had a major impact upon the theory and practice of management in this country's largest corporations, the impact upon mid-sized and small businesses has been marginal. Perhaps the main reason for this is that large corporations have the financial and personnel resources available to experiment with new ideas, while smaller organizations simply do not have the venture capital.

When compared with organizations in other economic sectors, most health care organizations are considered small to medium sized. The number of truly large organizations in the field is limited to the Hospital Corporation of America, Humana, American Medical International, National Medical Enterprises, and a few others. It is understandable then that health care organizations have not been the primary locus for Japanese management techniques and quality circles.

What does this mean for health care supervisors? The direct, simple meaning is that most health care supervisors will not have the chance to implement a quality circle program. The opportunity will not be there, because actual quality circles will not flourish within the limits of a single department. Their very nature requires strong support from top management. In practice, it is difficult to imagine top management giving sufficient support to a single department to develop a strong quality circle program.

However, progressive, supportive health care supervisors should not be disheartened if their organizations have not endorsed such new efforts. Health care supervisors first need to understand the reasons why their management does not initiate a quality circle program. Then, they must take the necessary steps to enhance employee participation within their areas of responsibility.

Reasons for lack of top management support

Health executives are under tremendous pressure to contain health care costs. Board members, third party payers, business coalitions, consumer groups, labor unions, government agencies, and other organizations are bombarding health administrators with demands to limit the increase in health care expenditures that have been rising rapidly for 20 years. Never before have health executives faced such a concerted challenge.

In this environment, a program usually has to have immediate bottom line benefits to an organization if it is to be accepted. Often, quality circles do not meet this test in the view of the organization's top decision makers.

Although some quality circle programs claim financial benefit within a few months, quality circles essentially offer an organization long-term gain. A major goal of these programs is to convince employees that their inputs have real meaning to organizations and that the quality circle program is not a fad that will be eliminated at the whim of executives.

Health care supervisors must realize that most executives, including health care executives, do not think that workers can significantly benefit their organizations beyond the direct output identified in an employee's job description. Most executives do not believe that giving employees a stake in the organization will reap benefits. There is no question that the ultimate goal of quality circles is to share decision making with workers.

To share decision making with workers is a democratic process. In essence, this means that executives must relinquish some of their existing authority and transfer that authority to workers. Among other considerations, the egos of a great many executives cannot handle the loss of authority because they see authority as being at the heart of management itself. For some, to transfer authority to workers would be analogous to taking out their own hearts.

Thus, the problem, in this dimension at least, is one of attitude rather than lack of knowledge or skills. As an individual's attitude triggers behavior, the outcome regarding the sharing of authority with workers meets resistance. Often this resistance is not communicated directly, because to do so would place the executive at risk. At the very least, it would be extremely embarrassing for most administrators to even imply that employees do not have the capacity to help the organization in ways other than the muscle needed to clean a floor.

Much more significant, however, is the fact that supporters of Japanese management, quality circles, and participative management have no absolute proof that their organizations will perform more effectively after implementing these programs. Supporters can state only that a preponderance of organizational behavior information from sociological and psychological studies indicates that employees will be more productive if management enables them to participate in decisions that affect their behavior in the work setting. That some managers buy into employee involvement principles means that this point of view has greatly influenced the attitudes of these managers. *Democratic managers* is the term that describes them.

An autocratic manager is not influenced to an appreciable extent by the argument advocating the inclusion of subordinates in organizational decision making. While strict autocrats are viewed in the 1980s as anachronistic, their numbers are still substantial. Among other considerations, they are not willing to take the organizational risk necessary to share decision making with workers.

What health care supervisors can do on their own

Some autocratic managers are in top management in health care organizations. Many simply would not support employee participation. Essentially, their view of the working world will not tolerate modern democratic thrusts. What can health care supervisors do who support employee involvement and would like to have the organization seriously consider Japanese management principles and quality circles?

What can health care supervisors do who support employee involvement and would like to have the organization seriously consider Japanese management principles and quality circles?

First, realize that Japanese management and quality circles are tools to use in the course of developing opportunities for workers in organizational decision making. By themselves, Japanese management and quality circles are not critical issues. While they are not fads, neither are they issues that divide good and bad supervisors or good and bad organizations. Simply, for American organizations and supervisors, they are steps away from uncaring, dictatorial management toward employee-supportive management. The critical issue is subordinate participation.

Second, take the initiative to do what you can within your sphere of responsibility to show all who care to observe, particularly the employees themselves, that you value worker participation and believe that workers have a role in decision making. Health care supervisors may be hesitant on their own to develop vehicles of employee participation in an organizational environment that is perceived as autocratic. However, superiors, regardless of style, usually appreciate supervisors who manage high quality departments regardless of their style. Thus, supervisors often have more latitude in their operations than they realize. Supervisors must remember that their superiors, particularly if they are at the executive level, have many other concerns, such as physicians, board members, and public officials. Most superiors want the supervisor to accomplish assigned and implied responsibilities and do not devote much time to reviewing the methods the supervisor uses to accomplish those responsibilities, so long as the methods are ethical. There is no question about the ethics of employee participation. Use windows of opportunity and involve workers.

Finally, take every opportunity to communicate your thinking about worker participation. Talk with peers and supervisors about what you think can be accomplished. If you are known as an effective health care supervisor, chances are that your influence in the organization is much greater than you suspect.

SUGGESTED READINGS

Cornell, L. "Quality Circles: A New Cure for Hospital Dysfunctions." *Hospital and Health Services Administration* 29 (September/October 1984): 88–93.

Goldstein, S.G. "Organizational Dualism and Quality Circles." *Academy of Management Review* 10 (1985): 504–17.

Keys, J.B., and Miller, T.R. "The Japanese Management Theory Jungle." *Academy of Management Review* 9 (1984): 342–53.

McKinney, M.M. "The Newest Miracle Drug: Quality Circles in Hospitals." *Hospital and Health Services Administration* 29 (September–October 1984): 74–87.

Munchus, G. "Employer–Employee Based Quality Circles in Japan: Human Resource Policy Implications for American Firms." *Academy of Management Review* 8 (1983): 255–61.

Ouchi, W. *Theory Z*. Reading, Mass.: Addison–Wesley, 1981.

"Quality: The U.S. Drives to Catch Up." *Business Week* (November 1, 1982): 66–69.

Shortell, S.M. "Theory Z: Implications and Relevance for Health Care Management." *Health Care Management Review* 7 (Fall 1982): 7–21.

Smith, H.L., and Burchell, R.C. "Japanese Management: Implications for Healthcare Administration." *Hospital and Health Services Administration* 29 (March–April 1984): 72–83.

Smith, R.L. "Theory Z: A Critical Analysis." *Arizona Business* 2 (second quarter 1983): 19–24.

Sullivan, J.J. "A Critique of Theory Z." *Academy of Management Review* 8 (1983): 132–42.

Yang, C.Y. "Demystifying Japanese Management Practices." *Harvard Business Review* 62 (November–December 1984): 172–82.

Yokl, R.T. "The Art of Japanese Management: Three Lessons to be Learned." *The Health Care Supervisor* 3 (October 1984): 80–86.

Quality control circles: A supervisor's tool for solving operational problems in nursing

F. Theodore Helmer
Associate Professor
College of Business Administration
Northern Arizona University
Flagstaff, Arizona

Sarath Gunatilake
Associate Professor
Health Science Department
California State University
Long Beach, California

QUALITY CONTROL circles, or QC circles as the Japanese call them, have received a strong burst of interest from managers throughout the world after the successful adoption of the technique in America in 1973. Today, numerous organizations are making use of QC circles to solve problems, improve quality, enhance productivity, and build employee morale. There is little documentation on the application of this technique to health care. However, the successful application of this technique might be one solution to the problem of nurses leaving the profession saying that management does not listen to them. This article discusses the successful implementation of QC circles in nursing services at several hospitals, some lessons learned, and the potential for increased application in hospitals throughout the world.

Health Care Superv, 1988, 6(4), 63–71
© 1988 Aspen Publishers, Inc.

BACKGROUND OF QUALITY CONTROL CIRCLES

The concept of QC circles was brought from Japan in the early 1970s when the United States began to study records of impressive productivity improvements achieved by the Japanese. At the time when the Japanese were experiencing their great industrial success, many nations found themselves in difficult circumstances. For example, between 1947 and 1967 the productivity of American workers grew at an average annual rate of only 3.1%, and during the last decade their productivity growth fell to 1.5% per year.

As perplexed managers and scholars sought answers to their productivity problems, they began to examine the success of the Japanese. In particular, research focused on the Japanese knack of utilizing the creativity of small work groups to improve productivity and product quality. It was discovered that Japanese managers appeared to be strong by making commitments to developing the skills of their employees fully, with the recognition that the employees had an important contribution to make to the organization's goals. The Japanese manager views the employees as resources that can be cultivated and utilized creatively to yield economic returns. This view sharply contrasts to the dominant ideology of western management, which has been largely inclined to discount worker cooperation and motivation in the improvement of productivity. In America, managers tend to assume that increased efficiency comes from better management, better technology, and greater capital investment, and not so much from worker commitment or motivation.

At the heart of these assumptions lies the perceived adversarial relationship between workers and management. The typical formal system of rules, job descriptions, supervision, grievances, and informal work practices reflects a lack of trust between the two groups and fosters the perception that the interests of the workers and the management are diametrically opposed. Management often acts as though it believes sincere worker cooperation is impossible to achieve.

In the early 1970s, a major U.S. study supported by the Department of Health, Education, and Welfare reported that the most consistent complaint of American workers was the failure of their superiors to listen to them when they were prepared to propose better ways of doing their jobs. "Workers feel that their bosses demonstrate little respect for their intelligence; superiors are said to perceive the workers as incapable of thinking creatively about their jobs."[1]

The comparison of management in the United States and Japan reveals numerous exceptions, yet it captures the different assumptions of managers in the two countries. When U.S. researchers visited Japan in the early 1970s, they found that quality control circles had literally become a national movement within industry, involving one out of every eight Japanese employees.[2]

A QC circle is a small group of employees doing similar or related work that meets regularly to identify, analyze, and solve product quality and production problems and to improve general operations. The ideal circle size is thought to be about ten, and the circle meets for an hour once a week. The circle leader asks the circle members to identify the problems to be addressed.

Management and staff can also recommend problems, but the decisions as to which problems to solve are left entirely to the discretion of the membership. The circle then selects a problem to be solved and conducts a formal problem analysis. Assistance can be sought from appropriate technical experts as well. Having analyzed the problem, and after arriving at a number of possible solutions, the circle makes its recommendations directly to management, usually by conducting a formal manage-

---

Quality control circles have proven their potential in health care as an effective tool for improving the quality of patient care, increasing employee job satisfaction, reducing costs, and maximizing productivity.

---

ment presentation. In principle, participation in a circle is voluntary, but in many Japanese organizations there is both peer and management pressure to join. The broader significance of the QC circle movement is utilization of education, experience, and creativity in the work force to help in planning and improvement, as well as improvement in worker morale.

When the story of QC circles was first disclosed outside of Japan, the reaction was one of astonishment, admiration, and envy. There were many questions and much discussion, all concerned with "How can a similar movement be created in my country?" Over the 20 years since the disclosure, there has been an explosion in the use of QC circles throughout the world. However, only a disappointingly small number of such

circles have been created in hospitals and health care organizations.[3]

In health care today and particularly in nursing in the western world, increased pressure exists to reduce costs at a time when nurses' values are changing. There is a dramatic change in nurses' expectations of how they should be treated and what role they can play in the organizations that employ them.[4] When these expectations are not met, nurses often become disenchanted, frustrated, and nonproductive. Today, nurses are demanding a high level of responsibility and an opportunity to be more participative, and they want greater participation with the medical staff in decision making. Since nursing service can represent as much as 60% of the hospital budget, these changing value systems must be recognized, understood, and integrated into the economic climate. At the same time, the hospital management system should fully involve nurses in its attempt to maximize productivity and reduce costs. Today, the trend is toward a more participative style of nursing management that involves nurses in work-related decisions and gives them a channel for making changes that will improve operations. A recent study of magnet hospitals reiterated the issue raised by staff nurses that nobody listens to them.[5] QC circles offer a system for nurses to be heard and to address problems and issues that they want to address.

QC circles have proven their potential in health care as an effective tool for improving the quality of patient care, increasing employee job satisfaction, reducing costs, and maximizing productivity. They involve nurses in decision making and facilitate communication among nursing staff, medical staff, and administration. This article describes in some detail how QC circles function, and relates the authors' experiences in conducting QC circle programs within a number of hospital settings.

QUALITY CONTROL CIRCLE OBJECTIVES

The implementation of any QC circle program begins with establishing and agreeing on objectives. In nursing, the bottom-line objective is one of cost reduction, with a variety of other subobjectives such as

- reduced nursing turnover,
- improved nursing staff morale,
- greater efficiency of operations,
- more effective scheduling,
- reduced absenteeism,
- improved quality of care,
- improved communications,
- more accurate cost allocation,
- reduced costs of patient care delivery, and
- improved nurse–physician relations.

Establishing objectives is a key step in the QC process and serves a number of purposes. These purposes include providing a solid foundation for gaining management support for the concept, selecting guidelines for the problem identification phase of each circle, and establishing a baseline against which the program's success can be evaluated.

Once specific objectives are established for the hospital, they are presented to administration for approval. For QC circles to be even possible, administration must have a sincere commitment and a high level of involvement and support. Most circles fail because of lack of sincere administrative support. If only lip service is provided, if

midmanagers feel their power is being undermined, and if top administration attempts to manipulate groups, then QC circles will probably not succeed. If the QC circle process is undertaken, it is extremely important that this be done with a total commitment to working toward success. Without this commitment the circles are bound to fail and will only foster an atmosphere of distrust and suspicion.[6]

Successful circles are found in hospitals where there is a strong belief in participatory management. All persons involved must believe that each employee or staff member of the hospital is an important and potentially useful resource. It is important, therefore, that circles be allowed to identify the problems they feel are important within their jurisdiction, free from undue pressure from administration. If administration starts and stops circles at its own discretion, rather than allowing circle members to make such decisions, the circles will not succeed. If administration dictates the problems, sets deadlines, or establishes specific cost savings, the process is bound to fail. Administration needs to realize that, in the initial stages, the circles will not be particularly productive as they work out their individual gripes and get the feel of how circle members mesh as a group. Administration needs to be patient during this period and not demand immediate results. Once this growing stage is completed, the circles can then work positively on problem solving. It is important for everyone to realize that the establishment of QC circles is a long-term project and a process, and not just a short-term attempt to solve an immediate problem. If the circle is considered only as a mechanism for solving a particular problem here and now, the potential of the approach as a preventive, dynamic, brainstorming, and problem-solving process is overlooked.

MAKING QUALITY CONTROL CIRCLES WORK

QC circles are groups of 7 to 12 employees from the same unit or department who meet regularly (usually once a week) to identify, analyze, and recommend solutions to work-related problems. Membership must be voluntary so that nursing staff does not feel manipulated (and, therefore, resentful) or coerced and threatened into membership. It may be very tempting to "pick the best" or "pick the people we know will do a good job," but such selection of members must be avoided as it can create suspicion about the validity and integrity of the circle and its members.

The key to successful QC circles is good planning and well-thought-through implementation. Questions that must be answered are (1) Is administration genuinely committed? (2) Have goals and objectives been clearly stated? (3) Has action been taken to establish a broad base? and (4) Have key persons been identified and trained?

A steering committee is a critical element to the success of the program. The steering committee consists of a group of key individuals selected from among management, circle leaders, and members. This committee is involved in making policy decisions and deciding on other details about planning, implementing, and evaluating the entire circle program. Since the committee defines program goals and policy, it is important that such a committee has full understanding of what quality circles are and how they operate. Otherwise, the committee may

inadvertently change a program design element without understanding the seriousness of its action. For example, attempts to introduce management by objectives (MBO) have failed in many situations because individuals assume that MBO means meeting all objectives and that the inability to meet any single objective as originally stated means failure. This type of lack of understanding of the concept results in the entire process becoming a farce and a frustrating experience for those who participate. It is important, therefore, that all those involved in planning and developing the QC circle process fully understand the concept.

In the event that the hospital has a labor union, the union stewards should be invited to participate in the leadership training program. This will help reduce the possible suspicion that productivity improvement means more work for less pay. Failure to inform the union may give the impression that efforts are being taken to circumvent and avoid the union in a management–labor issue. Historically, when unions have been involved in the process, the success of QC circles has been good because the unions soon found that the circles benefit their members. In cases in which unions have not been involved, circles have generally failed.

QC circles should be made clearly visible within the hospital. A modest but extensive internal public relations effort should be undertaken to let the staff know what QC circles are all about. This action is often overlooked as the organization focuses its efforts on getting the circles started. Such public relations efforts are critical, however, in that it is difficult to gain cooperation for a project when people do not know about it or do not understand it. Therefore, serious consideration must be given to this task.

The final step is to ensure that the circle selects a competent facilitator. A facilitator is responsible for coordinating the activities of a number of quality circles. This person's other roles include (1) creating and maintaining an open supportive atmosphere within each circle, (2) serving as a resource person to the circle, (3) training circle leaders and supervising member training, and (4) acting as liaison between the circle and management. It is important that the facilitator have the respect of hospital staff and have the people skills as well as the organizational skills needed to develop and implement quality circles within the hospital. This means that one of the best people in the hospital should be selected for this position rather than someone who has nothing else to do. To give credibility to the program and also to reflect administrative support, the facilitator should report directly to the chief administrator.[7]

TYPICAL EXPERIENCES WITH NURSING QUALITY CIRCLES

The authors have had extensive experience with more than 40 QC circles in a number of hospitals. The following scenarios are typical of these experiences.

Mountain View Hospital intensive care unit

A QC circle was initiated at the request of the members of the unit after the QC concept was presented in a routine supervisory management course. The nurses became excited about the possibilities and petitioned management to try out a circle for a short period. The meeting time was the shift changeover hour (3:30 P.M.), and meetings were held only if intensive care unit (ICU) census allowed. Ultimately, this circle developed an in-house registry, generating an estimated annual savings of more than $100,000. This circle enjoys a great deal of enthusiasm and management support and has been highly effective. The prime difference between this circle and the others mentioned below is the complete support and encouragement provided it by the director of nursing.

Central Clinic

At Central Clinic, one physician complained that his productivity was being impaired by an inefficient, uncooperative nursing staff embroiled in petty problems. A routine investigation of this four-physician specialty clinic included a study of patient flow, office layout, and scheduling systems. This revealed some minor problems but seemed to miss the major one. Discussions with the nursing supervisor revealed a 200% turnover in the staff of nine (four RNs, one LPN, two aides, and two unit clerks) during the previous 12 months. Interviews with each staff member confirmed that there was much mistrust and a general lack of motivation. It was decided to form a QC circle to define the key problems and select the ones to be addressed first.

At the first meeting, held over lunch, the role of QC circles was discussed, and group members were acquainted with the process. All were "volunteers," but there was a great deal of peer pressure to join. With an outsider as facilitator, there was an initial lack of trust and skepticism on the part of some circle members. Consequently, the early sessions were devoted to discussions of motivation, communication, perceptions, leadership, patient expectations, physician expectations, and trends in health care.

Circle members were encouraged to redefine their roles within the work unit and to provide constructive feedback regarding each other's behavior. After seven sessions of team-building preliminaries, the barriers to effective communication were broken down, and the members came together as a cohesive group and began circle activities in accordance with accepted procedures. They first discussed the numerous problems that the circle might address, and finally agreed on office and clinic layout as the place to start. It then took six additional circle meetings to review alternatives, implement changes, and recommend and finally evolve a new design. This new arrangement included additional shelves, better visibility into the waiting room, redesigned nurse work situations, new message boxes for physicians, and repositioning of the aides' stations. During this period of teamwork, morale and cooperation improved within the unit as staff members worked together to solve their common problems. Even a skeptical clerk who joined the group under intense peer pressure became an enthusiastic participant.

The group next addressed medical records flow, the system of calling in prescriptions, utilization of the examining room, labor work scheduling, and work assignments. These problems were addressed one at a time over the subsequent nine months. During that period not one staff member left the unit. Physician complaints disappeared as the average number of patients seen per day at the clinic increased by 4.2 with no apparent loss of quality.

Some of the innovations developed by the circle included a department motto of "concerned, quality care" along with a sign showing each staff member's name, a flexible appointment system to allow for walk-ins, joint use of examining rooms, better records management for return patients, and better physician–nurse communications. During a series of special QC meetings, each physician met with the group to discuss the latest technology in his or her field, the physician's methods of treatment, special surgical procedures, and other topics. The staff warmly welcomed these meetings—an added dimension that created a feeling of unity and a sense of teamwork that greatly improved morale, unit identity, and the quality of patient care.

Even a skeptical clerk who joined the group under intense peer pressure became an enthusiastic participant.

The foregoing process was no panacea; numerous problems were encountered and had to be resolved. There was no meeting time when all staff were available other than lunch; the QC meetings were brown bag meetings. At a unionized facility, the use of the lunch period would have been highly objectionable. The telephones and reception area had to be covered by float personnel during the meetings, at much inconvenience to the organization. The meeting day required some sacrifice in the number of patients seen just prior to the meeting, a measurable cost to the clinic but one that was judged to be a good investment. Significantly, this group dealt with issues of trust and interpersonal relationships before embarking on technical problem solving. A number of QC groups have failed that followed many QC manuals to the letter and jumped at once into technical problem solving without resolving the preliminary issues related to trust, leadership, and group maintenance.

LESSONS LEARNED FROM NURSING QUALITY CONTROL CIRCLES

From the foregoing experiences come several lessons:

- The potential for QC circles in health care is almost unlimited. No circle had any difficulty identifying problems for investigation. In the 40 circles with which the authors were extensively involved as facilitators, the average number of potential problems defined during the first circle meeting was 17.
- Management support is absolutely essential; it cannot be just a nod of the head. Management must be solidly behind the circle, and the use of a facilitator is highly recommended to keep this liaison with management.
- Physician support is paramount. If physicians do not see the need to improve nursing functions and do not want nurses in meetings for short periods of time, the concept cannot work. The nurse is trained to be responsive to the physician in the joint care of patients. If the physician does not communicate expectations to the nursing staff that include overall nursing efficiency, productivity, and effectiveness, there is no sense in starting up any circle involving nurses.
- No time pressures should be put on the circle for solutions, nor should man-

agement try to influence the circle's choice of problems to be analyzed.
- The union, if there is one, must be advised early in the development of circles and its cooperation must be sought. The union representative should be encouraged to join the circle as a member, not just as an observer. If the union chooses not to participate, it should be invited to each management presentation. Inclusion of unions has been favorable, although the unions were usually against the concept at the start.
- Overtime should be paid for circle meetings if they occur after hours. This is clearly where management should show its support.
- The lack of a convenient meeting time should not become an overwhelming obstacle. The concept of QC must be sold first. If people really want to meet, a time can always be found.
- Publicity helps after success. A little recognition can go a long way to encourage the circle to even greater results.
- Meetings should be limited to one hour, with tasks assigned for completion between meetings. Interruptions must be held to a minimum, and beepers or pagers should be discouraged.

●　　　●　　　●

The QC circle, as part of a nursing organization, is an exciting concept. It requires a dynamic, progressive director of nursing or other administrator to champion its introduction into the hospital. The potential payoffs are great; experience shows that a better hospital and a more highly motivated nursing staff will result. The cost is minimal. The authors sincerely hope that these expe-riences will motivate nursing administrators to start quality circles in their hospitals to enhance nursing, the patients, and the insti-tution.

REFERENCES

1. U.S. Department of Health, Education, and Welfare. *A Profile of American Workers*. Report HEW 72018. Washington, D.C.: Government Printing Office, April 1972.
2. Yager, E.G. "The Quality Circle Explosion." *Training and Development Journal* 35, no. 4 (1981): 89–99, 101–05.
3. Ibid.
4. Wine, J.A. and Baird, J.E., Jr. "Improving Nursing Management and Practice through Quality Circles." *Journal of Nursing Administration* 13, no. 5. (May 1983): 5–10.
5. American Academy of Nursing, Task Force on Nursing Practice in Hospitals. *Magnet Hospitals: Attraction and Retention of Professional Nurses*. Kansas City, Mo.: ANA, 1983.
6. Helmer, F.T. "Quality Circle Applications in Nursing." *Quality Circle Digest* 2, no. 5 (1982): 15-21.
7. Gunatilake, S. "An Exploratory Study of Quality Circles and Team Building in Two Hospital Settings." Ph.D. diss., School of Public Health, University of Hawaii, 1984.

Involving employees in change, productivity and the future

William B. Werther, Jr.
Professor of Management
College of Business
  Administration
Arizona State University
Tempe, Arizona

HEALTH CARE organizations are in the forefront of change, and supervisors in this environment are continually forced to experiment with innovative work place arrangements—from new procedures to new technologies. These changes will extend well beyond scheduling adjustments to entire new patterns of managing. As the rate of change accelerates, much of the impact will be felt by first-level supervisors. How nonsupervisory employees react to these changes will shape the success, reputation and future of many health care supervisors and their employers.

A variety of identifiable factors virtually guarantee that waves of change will confront the health care industry. Four of the major forces that ensure change are rising costs, demographics, technology and the demand for health care. Cost increases stem from many sources. General inflation, new technologies, expansion, supplies

Health Care Superv, 1984,2(2),1–14
© 1984 Aspen Publishers, Inc.

and salaries are but a few of these sources. Neither boards of directors nor regents can influence many of these cost factors, with the noteworthy exception of labor costs. Most costs are largely fixed. However, with ongoing pressure from governments and other third party payers to restrain costs further, health care providers will face additional pressures to become more productive. External pressure on top managements will translate into direct pressure on supervisors to make their work groups more productive.

Cost containment and productivity improvement are closely intertwined. Labor cost—a major expense item in most health care budgets—offers a prime example. Often advances in wages and benefits are assumed to increase labor costs directly, and usually this relationship holds. However, increases in labor costs are determined by increases in wages and benefits minus any gains in productivity.

When productivity does not change and wages or benefits increase by, for example, 5 percent, labor costs can rise by up to 5 percent as well. If, however, wages and benefits go up by 5 percent and productivity improves by 3 percent, actual labor costs can rise by no more than 2 percent. Should productivity improve even faster than wages and benefits, labor costs actually decline—a most unusual situation in any organization. Thus employee demands for higher wages and benefits are compatible with pressures for lower or stable

> *If wages and benefits go up by 5 percent and productivity improves by 3 percent, actual labor costs can rise by no more than 2 percent.*

costs *only* if productivity improvement occurs. Inevitably, pressures for cost containment in health care will mean additional efforts aimed at productivity improvement.

Demographic changes in both the work force and the general population also will add impetus for productivity improvement. The declining birth rate of the 1960s and 1970s means that the growth of the labor force will slow throughout the 1980s and into the 1990s. Assuming even modest economic growth during the next decade, skilled help will become increasingly scarce. Those with needed skills will be vigorously sought by other segments of the economy. Shortages among skilled professionals and technicians will place additional pressure on supervisors to find innovative methods of increasing productivity.

Future changes in the population also create a need for improved productivity. As the average age of the population increases, the demand for health services will increase. Particularly rapid growth will be experienced in nursing homes and other types of extended care facilities. Here again, the increased demand will be met with new facilities, procedures and equipment. However, the need for hands-on care must be met at least partially by increased productivity, especially in geographic areas in which shortages of skilled practitioners become apparent as the growth in the work force slows.

When cost pressures, declining labor availability and increased demand face most industries, the classic response is for firms to merge in search of economies of scale. The resulting larger scale employers use even greater amounts of capital and labor-saving automation. To some extent, the health care industry is responding in the classic manner, as evidenced by the growth of proprietary and nonprofit chains of hospitals, nursing homes and other health care facilities. Likewise, increases in applied technology and automation are apparent in some laboratories, clinics and records sections. However, the ability to geographically centralize health care facilities is limited by the need to put facilities near to their users. Automation and technology are further limited in those activities in which hands-on care is required. In short, health care employers are severely limited in their ability to centralize, automate or outbid other industries for talent. At the same time, pressures exist to lower costs while the demand for health care increases and the labor market grows at a decreasing rate.

THE PEOPLE OPTION

People—blue collar and white collar alike—are the key to any cost control effort. Admittedly, better equipment utilization, occupancy rates and financial controls can help, but each of these and other approaches are controlled by the people in the organization. If every person is fully committed to improving his or her contribution to the organization, the result will be improved productivity. That is, more fully dedicated people can produce more laboratory tests, more filed records, more nursing care or increased amounts of other outcomes during their shifts. Even modest increases in effort can lead to substantial gains in organizational productivity. In turn, higher levels of productivity make the facility more efficient and better able to provide quality health care at minimum cost. Restated, improved productivity means better service at lower costs.

Obviously, the organization, its supervisors and its clients or patients will benefit. However, nonsupervisory employees seldom sense any benefit for themselves in improving productivity. Productivity increases usually mean simply that they work harder. Even worse, higher productivity may be seen as bringing layoffs or at least unwanted reassignments.

The health care supervisor is likely to be caught in the middle between top management pressure for more productivity and employee resistance to "working harder." Effective supervisors cannot realistically expect top management to retreat from its urgent need for greater productivity. External pressures, often coupled with personal career ambitions, are simply too strong. The supervisor's best hope is to reduce employee resistance to work place innovations aimed at increasing productivity. But how can supervisors reduce resistance to change?

Resistance to change

It is axiomatic that people do not resist their own ideas. If a person has an idea that he or she believes is a good one, resistance to it is unthinkable because the person "owns" the idea. "Ownership" of an idea creates pride in it. The "owner" wants to see the idea grow and flourish because with a "healthy" idea its originator can probably make his or her job easier and better. If others see the merit in the idea, recognition of the owner often follows and pride is the likely outcome.

To the extent that a supervisor can create a sense of ownership in productivity improvement among employees, changes are less likely to be resisted. In fact, supervisors who are the most successful at creating a sense of ownership find that employees actually view change as a normal, even integral, part of their job. These same employees also see themselves as change agents—people who suggest and facilitate change.

The key to creating this type of climate in an organization centers around employee participation in the decision-making process. Employee participation does not mean that employees are involved in every decision, nor does it mean that employees are involved with decisions that do not affect them. Janitors do not suddenly vote on the purchase of X-ray equipment, and nurses do not decide on surgical procedures. However, janitors *do* have legitimate input to provide to those decisions that concern the purchase of cleaning supplies and equipment; nurses *do* have the capacity to consult with physicians about patients' courses of treatment.

Some supervisors create resistance to change by the way they supervise. Often by observing other managers or former supervisors, they incorrectly assume that they are there solely to make decisions. Their style is to gather the facts, review the alternatives and decide. Then the "fun" begins; resistance to change occurs because those affected by the decision feel they had no part in the decision-making process. They have no ownership of the decision. They can take little pride in success or feel little responsibility for failure. If the decision requires more or new efforts—as many decisions do—employees see real costs but see no corresponding benefits. Even with a good "sales job" by the supervisor, employees are likely to be less than enthusiastic about the changes brought on by the supervisor's decision.

The distinction that is sometimes missed by supervisors (and their managers) is that they assume that managers are paid to make decisions. Except under the rarest of circumstances, members of management are not paid to make decisions but rather are paid to get decisions made. Their role is to facilitate the correct actions. If a decision is needed, those affected by the decision should participate in its formulation and resolution. Then—and only then—can a supervisor expect resistance to change to be minimized. Even when a supervisor is given a directive by higher management, employee involvement in the methods to be used to implement the directive can help create some ownership and lessen resistance to change.

In dealing with resistance to change, supervisors face a hierarchy of solutions. At the top of the list is involvement because, as explained above, it dissolves resistance before it builds by creating ownership among those who are affected since they are involved in the decision-making process.

At the next level is the need to "sell" employees. Here the supervisor attempts to overcome resistance to change by "selling" the idea to employees. This approach may work in some cases, but when it does succeed, it seldom generates enthusiastic support. At best, those affected acquiesce to the change. They do not support it actively but neither do they actively resist it. This "sales approach" often fails because the supervisor focuses his or her sales arguments on the reasons why the change is needed. The reasons may be valid and the logic impeccable, but these rational reasons often overlook the emotional or feeling side of the decision.

If the employees feel that the idea is being sold too hard, if they feel it is not in their best interest, if they feel their ideas are not considered, if they feel a better way exists, if they feel the change is unwarranted, if they feel aggrieved by some other management action, then they may reject the "sales pitch." Supervisory laments about the "logic" of their position or that "employees should" accept the decision are so much hot air. If the sales pitch is not congruent with employee emotions, it probably will fail. Even if it "succeeds" passive acceptance is more likely than active support.

What the supervisor is faced with is to issue a direct order. This final approach of "telling" employees may work. Employees may do what they are told. Or they may resist by refusing or by sabotaging the decision. Sabotage may be likely not because the employees are "bad" in any fundamental sense, but because they need to assert their "rights" or their identity. Should the employees refuse, supervisory credibility is damaged, sometimes severely and permanently, with the work group. Telling employees is often a last resort of supervisors who have failed to consider the emotional impact of their decisions.

Future patterns of management

For the "people option" to be played out, the organizational climate in most health care settings must become more receptive to employee

> *Creation of a receptive climate is the responsibility of every member of management. It takes hard work.*

ideas. Creation of a receptive climate is the responsibility of every member of management. It takes hard work. Top-level managers obviously exert broad influence on the organizational climate. They cannot expect to tap the creativity of all employees with simple memos or directives. Top managers must create such a climate by using their leadership style as an example; they must actively solicit advice from those they supervise. Pseudoparticipation (in which the manager has already decided and is merely using involvement until someone "discovers" the right answer) or manipulative participation (in which the purpose of involvement is to avoid resistance to change rather than to foster a true, collective investigation of the problem, its options and its implementation) are probably worse than an honest, primitive, dictatorial style. However, without a move toward a more open, participative style by top management, it is unlikely, and even unreasonable, to expect supervisors to use a more open style.

Although no one style fits all supervisors and not all situations deserve the same supervisory style, some styles seem to create work place "culture" that is more receptive to change. Autocratic styles often treat employ-ees as "children," in a transactional sense. Workers are told what to do, with little room allowed for employee ideas. This approach assumes the employee cannot or will not make a contribution. Excluding emergency situations—such as a hospital emergency department—this approach may create resignations among those who are able to leave and apathy among those who stay.

Closely allied is the bureaucratic approach. Here the concern of the supervisor is to do what the procedures call for, which may or may not be the right thing to do. The mentality is one where the supervisor shows little initiative but instead seeks "safe" solutions, whether those solutions are appropriate or not.

A proactive, consultative approach is a style that generates greater support from employees. This style finds the supervisor looking for necessary changes to improve performance of the unit. By involving the employee, not only is resistance less likely, but the supervisor also gains the benefit of additional input that may help create a more optimal solution.

For those supervisors confident of their management abilities, a move toward more participative approaches can offer opportunities for less resistance and greater productivity, regardless of top management's style. However, if top management sets a tone, a climate, by its example, supervisors are much more likely to receive support for their participative efforts. Neither supervisors nor top managers can tap the wellspring of employee creativity with an order. Instead, systematic efforts are needed to create an organizational climate that is conducive to helping people find new and better ways of providing service.

Approaches to involvement

Since the people option is best tapped through employee involvement, more and more top managements are moving toward supporting efforts aimed at greater participation of employees in decision making. Experience among health care organizations and the business sector suggests several approaches that seem appropriate for health care settings.

Quality circles

Quality circles are groups of employees who meet with their common supervisor to identify and solve work-related problems. Usually the supervisor and his or her direct reporting staff meet for one hour per week as part of their usual shift or on an overtime basis. These meetings occur after the supervisor has received two or three full days of training on leadership, conducting meetings, group dynamics and problem solving. The supervisor's employees usually receive one day of training in various problem-solving techniques.

During their weekly meetings, at which attendance of employees is voluntary, problems of concern to the entire group are identified and discussed. The problem that emerges as the group's "consensus" pick is in-

vestigated before the next meeting. At the second meeting additional discussion is conducted, followed by additional data gathering the following week. The cycle is repeated until the group identifies the causes of the problem and develops its solution. If the solution is within the supervisor's authority, the group's solution is implemented. Otherwise, the circle members make a presentation to the appropriate level of management to secure authorization to make the changes necessary to eliminate the problem.

Since membership in the circle is voluntary and the decision-making process is participative, the results of the group's deliberations are not "management's decision." Instead, all members of the group "own" the problem and its solution.

Perhaps more noteworthy is the process of discussing problems faced by the group and identifying solutions. This process leads to a higher level of quality of work life. Even employees who have boring, repetitive jobs may now have the chance to help shape their work environment. Attitudes, morale and communications all improve. These benefits made through the circle meetings carry over to the group's regular activities during the rest of the work week. Also, since work place problems are solved, productivity goes up. Although circles can fail—particularly if the leader runs them autocratically or management does not act on the circles' recommendations—circles that continue to meet week after week can be assumed to be successful on some level or the volunteer members would most likely have quit.

For supervisors, circles mean additional training and they mean the supervisor must be receptive to employee ideas. The supervisor remains the supervisor. Leadership responsibilities are not shared. What is shared is the excitement and frustration of the decision-making process.

Before "volunteering" to become involved in quality circles, the supervisor would do well to talk with his or her immediate supervisor. Why? Because, too often, top management may be convinced that quality circles are the "right way to go." They may then order up a task force to get, as one manager said, "some of those round, Japanese things started." Dutifully, the personnel department or the office of quality control starts up a half-dozen or more. Top management wants them, supervisors volunteer and are trained, members are trained, and the circles begin. Often they begin with some notable successes. However, middle-level managers— often the supervisor's direct superior—have not been consulted. Likewise, middle managers probably received no training or only a cursory "three-hour seminar."

After the circles have operated for a while, top management's pronouncements about the importance of quality circles fade in frequency and intensity. Middle-level managers who did not fully understand the nature of quality circles and who were not par-

ticularly committed to the concept in the first place, often begin to show less and less support for circle requests and "one-hour per week boondoggles." With middle-level management support declining, supervisors may find that they too begin to lose their enthusiasm for this useful management tool. In short, does your boss support quality circles because he or she believes in them, or are they supported because higher management finds circles to be the "in" fad?

Suggestion systems

Suggestion systems already exist in many health care facilities. However, in most facilities these suggestion programs work poorly, if at all. Nevertheless, some managements have revitalized their suggestion systems and have discovered a wealth of employee ideas that can improve productivity. These "new" or "revised" approaches rely heavily on supervisory involvement.

An employee's idea is first discussed with the supervisor. The idea is then reduced to writing, signed by the employee, and reviewed by the supervisor for accuracy and clarity. Even if the supervisor disagrees with the idea, the supervisor signs the suggestion to indicate his or her familiarity with it. The idea then goes to a central clearing office for assignment to a facility engineer or some other person in a position to evaluate the idea objectively. The resulting recommendation is communicated to the worker and supervisor. If the idea is approved, implementation follows. Otherwise, the employee is told why his or her idea was rejected.

The keys to this involvement approach seem to be two: supervisory receptivity and feedback. During informal discussions with the employee, a supervisor can often discourage an employee from "writing up the idea." Effective supervisors, however, "talk up" the need for employee ideas in an effort to create a positive environment for the creation of ideas.

Immediate feedback is essential. The average suggestion system takes approximately 80 days from the time the idea is first reduced to writing until the final evaluation is communicated to the employee. Truly effective systems provide the employee a response within a few weeks, sometimes within a few days.

The value of a suggestion system is easy to understand. Virtually any employee could suggest a better way to do his or her job. Even if the improvement was designed only to make the job easier, productivity improvement is likely to follow. Most changes that make a job easier make it more productive too. Even if the idea is a change that does not actually improve productivity, such as moving a desk away from the air vent to avoid a draft, it allows the employee to feel that he or she can have some influence on the organization. This feeling of influence can enhance the employee's feelings of satisfaction with the job and acceptance by the supervisor.

Even in the absence of a formal suggestion system, supervisory acceptance of employee ideas helps to create a more open environment in which employee–supervisor communications are characterized mainly as adult-to-adult transactions.

Communications

Perhaps the most fundamental approach to employee involvement is through communications. Few actions by supervisors make an employee feel more a part of the organization than learning about the organization, feeling on the "inside." Formal communications programs from monthly newspapers to daily newsletters on cafeteria tables all can help. Bulletin boards and payroll stuffers are useful as well. However, few communications channels can rival face-to-face communications with a person's supervisor.[1]

Perhaps the most fundamental approach to employee involvement is through communications.

The content of supervisory communications can shape the productivity and satisfaction found in the work place. Although social chitchat is useful for keeping communications channels open, of primary importance are communications that let the employee know what is going on in the organization. Changes in policies, procedures and personnel are obvious topics. One subject too often overlooked is the group's performance. In some departments, measures of results are commonly maintained. Orders filled in the pharmacy, laboratory tests run in the clinic or patients billed by bookkeeping are usual examples. In other areas—such as a nursing station—measures may be meaningless or even counterproductive. For example, a nurse's productivity cannot (and probably should not) be measured by the number of medications dispensed in any one shift, day or month. However, where accurate and usable measures of performance are kept, communicating these measures to those who are responsible is often an effective way of providing meaningful feedback that can enhance both productivity and quality of work life.

Perhaps no area of communications is more important than new employee orientation. The new health care worker arrives with a largely blank slate about the organization, except for the selection process, and a blank slate about the supervisor. It is at this point, called organizational entry, that a supervisor can have a profound effect on creating a viable communications link with the newcomer.

Time should be spent with the newcomer by giving him or her an orientation. The basics of any orientation include an introduction to the people, place, policies and performance associated with the job. People, perhaps, are the most important to the employee. Not only should the

introduction include name, title and job, but additional insights about each employee help the newcomer remember and relate to the often overwhelming rush of faces. For example, if the newcomer and an old-time employee have some common interest (hobbies), family status (a recent parent), education (degree or school) or other parallel between them, the supervisor can greatly accelerate the socialization process. Likewise, assigning a "buddy," a peer to help show the newcomer around, further solidifies social relationships. It helps the socialization process because the buddy will often introduce the new employee to his or her friends around the job site through invitations to lunch, coffee breaks or after-work activities.

The supervisor also should inform the newcomer about the place. Location of safety equipment, fire equipment, cafeteria and even rest rooms may be appropriate.

Of course, key policies should be explained. Given the "high need to please" that many new employees have, the supervisor has a never-to-be-repeated opportunity to emphasize key policies that are crucial to operating success.

Another important topic is performance expectations. If the supervisor conveys his or her confidence in the newcomer's potential, successful performance is likely. This Pygmalion effect may allow a supervisor to add to the newcomer's self-confidence during an uncertain time, the first few days on a new job. Not only will self-image-enhancing statements speed up the socialization process, but they can help develop a communications bond between the supervisor and the newcomer. At the same time, if the employee ends this orientation phase of organizational entry with high performance expectations, actual performance is more likely to be satisfactory in a shorter period. The speed-up in learning apparently occurs because the employee's "new job anxieties" are substantially reduced by a thorough orientation program. Even employees on routine, low-skilled jobs master those jobs faster when they receive an orientation that covers the people, place, policies and performance expectations of their new organization.

Experimenting with involvement

Whether quality circles, suggestion systems, improved communications or other approaches are used, employee involvement is likely to grow more common in health care. For many supervisors, it will be a major and increasing, if not necessarily new, force.

Experimental efforts by personnel departments, productivity administrators, top managers and individual supervisors are becoming more common. Not every approach is successful, but even the failures can help supervisors learn the limits of a more participative approach. When such approaches are used sincerely, employees often appreciate supervisors who attempt to consider their needs.

FORCES FOR PRODUCTIVITY IMPROVEMENT

Specific health care facilities and specific functions within those facilities will face different sources of pressure. Although more pressures for productivity improvement and the cost savings usually associated with it are likely in all health care settings, the degree of pressure and the rate of change will vary from organization to organization, with proprietary facilities often leading the way. Therefore, it is impossible to identify every force for productivity improvement that supervisors are likely to encounter. However, computers and other forms of automation, along with a gradual restructuring of some traditional health care jobs, are two broad forces likely to be experienced by all health care supervisors.

Computers and beyond

Time magazine's "Man of the Year" award was won by the computer in 1982. The significance of that selection should not be lost on health care supervisors. The use of computers will increase rapidly during the next few years. Some experts argue that we have not even entered the computer age any further than Edison entered the age of electricity. With the cost-to-performance ratio of computers continuing to fall while the capabilities of computers grow, the trend toward computerization of records and charts will continue. The major changes will likely be in "smart machines."

Robots that deliver and collect mail already are in use. Some housekeeping and orderly functions are likely to succumb to these smart machines. Perhaps the greatest impact of these machines will be to make diagnostic and analytical tools available close to the patient and operated by nurses or technicians. Portable, fast, electronic analyzers are likely to be accompanied by computer-controlled therapy equipment.

If these electronic marvels do indeed proliferate in availability as costs decline, the key impact on supervisors will be in training and overseeing those who use these new machines. Although some equipment will be self-explanatory (literally, through the use of voice synthesizers) and other equipment will be fully automated, the responsibility for the machine-to-patient interface is likely to remain with the operator and therefore ultimately with the operator's first-level supervisor.

Job restructuring

As computerization increases, systems analysts will think their way through many procedures. At the same time, personnel departments will report growing difficulties in meeting staffing needs, especially where hard-to-find professiona and technical skills are concerned. One likely outcome of these two forces may be a rather radical restructuring of many jobs.

Some of these trends are evident today. For example, a shortage of nurses can basically be overcome by increasing pay dramatically to attract nurses from other institutions or from other careers. To do so, of course, means upsetting internal pay scales and other associated costs. Instead, some hospitals are meeting the shortage by restructuring the nurse's job and assigning many traditional nursing functions to nonnurses. The intent is to free the nurse to do those activities for which only a nurse is qualified. Running errands, housekeeping chores and the like are being increasingly delegated. This trend is likely to be seen wherever highly trained technicians and professionals appear to be in short supply. Likewise, in laboratory, food service, housekeeping and records departments, hospital administrators are likely to undertake job restructuring as they add new equipment and procedures in search of higher productivity.

Shortages, surpluses and obsolescence

Computers, advanced equipment and job restructuring will resolve some human resource shortages, but shortages will still occur in many highly skilled areas of health care. Part of the response will be increased technical training by employers and third parties—such as universities, consultants and equipment vendors. In-house training is also likely to increase dramatically as a means of keeping up with the latest changes. All these changes, in turn, indicate a need for even more supervisory training in the future if health care supervisors are to avoid the trap of obsolescence.

At the same time, surpluses will occur. Advances in technology may be able to eliminate some jobs completely. These surplus jobs may first appear as health care growth slows— and, obviously, the growth will slow because at current growth rates half the U.S. population would be working in health care by the next century if double-digit growth rates continue. As growth slows and technology matures, advances in the business office, housekeeping, laboratory and other departments may mean a need for fewer people. "Doing more with less" is a practical definition of productivity. If big strides in labor productivity are to occur, supervisors will be expected to find ways to "do more with fewer people."

The press of technology-induced productivity means that supervisors will have to manage greater complexity and face greater diversity in their jobs. A subtle source of this complexity and diversity can be found among employees themselves. Prior to the 1970s, most employees had similar work-related values. Today the supervisor oversees those with "tradi-

---

The press of technology-induced productivity means that supervisors will have to manage greater complexity and face greater diversity in their jobs.

---

tional values" formed among people who established these values in the "golden era of radio." Another group might be labeled the "television generation." These post-World War II "babies" largely have been absorbed into the work force. As any supervisor knows, these two groups of workers vary, sometimes widely, in their attitudes toward organizational loyalty, overtime, authority and even work itself. Just starting to infiltrate health care organizations is a new wave of workers who are products of the computer age. This generation is nearly fearless of electronic technology— from video games to microcomputers—and possesses attitudes toward work that are different from the previous generations of workers. In coming years, health care supervisors will be supervising a blend of all three generations. Just the introduction of new technologies—technologies almost certain to come—will tax the creativity, patience and skill of even the most sophisticated supervisor.

The result? Uncertain. What is certain, however, is that the health care supervisor will face challenges, during the remainder of this century and into the next, greater than all the changes seen during the last 100 years. Although the technological changes seem the most obvious, the sociocultural expectations of workers and the pressures for productivity are likely to create the greatest clash—a clash more difficult to comprehend and resolve than the mere introduction of job-changing and people-threatening technologies.

TOWARD THE FUTURE

As health care institutions move toward the future, rapid and extensive change seems a certainty. This change will create growth and promotional opportunities for many health care supervisors. New challenges are likely to arise from the need to discover new ways to manage people. As the roles of health care practitioners grow more complex within an ever-increasingly complex environment, more and more of the burdens of change and productivity improvement will fall to the health care supervisor.

Those supervisors who seek to involve their employees in the decision-making process are much more likely to discover the cooperation, and even the active support, of those they supervise. Supervisors who are threatened by these changes and try to conceal their fears through autocratic decision making rather than more participative approaches are likely to find extensive changes met by extensive resistance. Their failure to implement needed changes, from new equipment to new procedures or job designs, may well mean personal and career failure and harm to their facilities' future productivity. Only through the involvement of employees are supervisors likely to earn the support needed to manage change, productivity and the future.

REFERENCE

1. D'Aprix, R. "The Oldest (and Best) Way to Communicate with Employees." *Harvard Business Review* 60 (September–October 1982): 30, 32.

Part IV
Other Dimensions of Productivity Improvement

Incentive compensation and the health care supervisor

Jerad D. Browdy
President
Jerad D. Browdy, Inc.
Evanston, Illinois

MANY CHANGES are occurring in the delivery of health care in the United States, but it is not the intent of this article to dwell on them. All health care professionals and managers are aware of the impact of mergers, acquisitions, competition, and alternative delivery systems on their jobs and careers. Some of the most profound changes affecting supervisors at all levels, however, are those occurring in health care management compensation practices. It is this single area of rapid change on which this article focuses.

Traditionally, health care compensation programs were basically egalitarian in nature. All persons in the organization received similar fringe benefits and pay increases. Even at the management level, annual increases were predicated on longevity rather than performance. However, this is changing rapidly, and longevity-based increases are being re-

Health Care Superv, 1987, 5(3), 43–54
© 1987 Aspen Publishers, Inc.

placed by pay-for-performance compensation systems. The most dramatic change in this area is the rapidly increasing interest in and implementation of performance-based management incentive compensation systems.

The full extent of the incentive approach to compensation can be seen in recent management salary surveys conducted among approximately 200 distinguished not-for-profit health care institutions in 30 states. Almost 25 percent of the participants have developed, or are in the process of developing, performance-based incentive systems for their management groups. A similar survey conducted in 1983 among essentially the same participants indicated less than 5 percent of the respondents had implemented incentive plans. The increase is dramatic but not especially surprising in light of current conditions.

Before discussing the impact of incentive compensation on the health care supervisor, the following reviews the primary reasons for the increasing interest in incentive compensation in general:

- Increasingly, health care executives and managers feel that the ability to maintain a fiscally viable and growing organization in spite of diagnosis related groups (DRGs), competition, and increasingly stringent cost containment measures requires compensation considerations beyond the traditional annual salary increase.

- Trustees are seeking executives and managers with entrepreneurial outlooks who are competitive and willing to take risks. These individuals are, in turn, perfectly willing to risk failure, but they expect to be compensated accordingly for their successes.

- Trustees, particularly those from the corporate sector, are beginning to insist that management salaries be based on quantifiable performance standards rather than longevity.

- As the dollars available for salary increases decline, trustees and chief executive officers are coming to recognize that there is a point beyond which the annual salary increase may no longer be feasible. This is particularly true for individuals paid in the upper quartiles of their salary ranges. However, trustees and chief executive officers are seeking ways to reward the achievers without continuing to increase base salaries annually. It is also being recognized that some spectacular achievements of a singular nature can best be rewarded by means other than salary increases.

- As not-for-profit health care organizations continue to establish for-profit affiliates it is becoming necessary to recruit managers from the business sector. The compensation expectations of these individuals may not be compatible with traditional health care management compensation programs.

There is some confusion with respect to the definition of incentive compensation. For example, the terms *performance bonus* and *incentive compensation* are frequently used synonymously. They are not the same, however, and the differences should be understood.

The performance bonus is, more often than not, highly subjective and based upon some past significant achievement that usually has not been predicted. Sometimes, a performance bonus is granted to all employees or to a segment of the employee population if the institution has had a particularly good fiscal year. This has often occurred in health care, but the award was usually small—a week's salary or so. However, an increasing number of institutions are beginning to award discretionary bonuses to their executives and managers based on significant, unpredicted achievements during the course of the year. Such rewards now frequently amount to several thousand dollars. In other words, some type of bonus is awarded based on a retrospective review of past performance.

Incentive compensation in the strictest sense, on the other hand, is usually based on the achievement of specific, quantifiable, predetermined objectives (targets) considered to be beyond the threshold of normal or expected job performance. This is the approach most commonly considered and implemented in health care today and the one having the most direct impact on supervisors. Fre-

quently, the previously mentioned performance bonus is the starting point in developing a true incentive system. While not an incentive system in the purest sense it may be an effective method for the management group to become accustomed to some bonus possibility based on specific performance levels.

A performance-based incentive plan should not be arbitrarily imposed on the management group.

A performance-based incentive plan should not be arbitrarily imposed on the management group. While the plan itself should be simple, there are a number of complex issues that should be addressed prior to the actual development of the plan's mechanics. It is critical that the following issues be addressed by those contemplating implementation of a plan for their organization.

- determine the philosophy and purpose of the plan;
- establish award criteria;
- identify the incentive-eligible group;
- establish administrative and control procedures; and
- decide on the appropriate type of plan.

Decisions made within the foregoing areas will obviously have a great impact on those executives and managers considered for inclusion in an incentive plan.

DETERMINING PURPOSE AND PHILOSOPHY

Basically, three questions must be addressed in determining purpose and philosophy for an incentive compensation program:

1. Is the plan intended to reward extraordinary achievement beyond the threshold of normal or expected job performance?
2. Is the plan actually the merit portion of the merit increase?
3. Is the plan intended to encourage teamwork and cooperation within the eligible group?

There are critical differences among the foregoing. The purpose of most incentive plans that are based on predetermined, quantifiable objectives is to reward extraordinary achievements beyond the expectation of normal job performance. There are some situations, however, in which the basic salary structure is not competitive, and incentives are used to bring compensation to a competitive level. Incentive compensation is *not* a substitute for a competitive base salary structure.

Point three is exceedingly important. Many chief executive officers view incentive compensation as an excellent means of encouraging cooperative efforts of the eligible group in striving to achieve specific corporate goals. This is realistic in an environment in which the management style is collegial and participatory. However, it can be disastrous in an environment in which the management style is politically charged and marked by intense personal competition within the management group. In this latter situation a highly individualized incentive plan may be desirable and effective.

ESTABLISHING AWARD CRITERIA

Establishing criteria for awarding performance is clearly the most critical phase of the incentive process. The primary concern to be addressed is exactly what is the institution paying for. It is the award criteria that can cause the most consternation among those responsible for developing the plan, and it is the award criteria that will generally determine the incentive-eligible group.

Why is the determination of award criteria a perplexing problem to those responsible for the incentive system design? In the business and industrial sector the basis for mangerial incentive awards is frequently predetermined profitability or net income goals (also return on investment, sales, or production targets). Incentive goals in terms of profitability, production market share, or sales are relatively easy to define.

A common perception among many health care managers is that specific, quantitative performance measurements are difficult to establish. It has been felt that state, federal, and even local regulatory restraints, beyond the control of the health care management group, affect the institution's management objective-setting practices.

Such perceptions are, and always have been, invalid. It is for these very reasons that health care institutions are beginning to recognize that incentive compensation must become a major element of the total management compensation program. The ability of the institution to survive, grow, and prosper in an increasingly competitive and complex environment is directly dependent upon the skills and talents of the management group. In simplistic terms, it is the efficient institutions that will be rewarded and in turn it will be the efficient managers who will be rewarded.

Within the context of cost constraints and competition, definitive objectives, usually fiscal in nature, are being imposed on management at all levels. This is a concept frequently misunderstood by health care supervisors. It is not unusual for supervisors, particularly those involved in direct patient care, to feel that a bottom-line emphasis on incentive targets will have an adverse effect on patient care. However, it must be recognized that the demands for cost containment and the competitive nature of the environment absolutely dictate that the institution be fiscally viable for institutional survival. The concern about a fiscally oriented incentive system is understandable, but there should be ample quality controls including the Joint Commission on Accreditation of Hospitals

(JCAH) and professional practice standards to ensure that quality is not compromised. This is a critical element of any incentive plan.

The next important question to consider is how incentive targets are established and who sets them. Ultimately, the incentive plan should be directly related to the institution's overall objective-setting process. It is not the intent of this article to dwell on objective setting, because it is a complex subject in and of itself. However, the objective-setting process should begin at the very top of the organization, with the trustees and chief executive officer defining the mission of the organization. A strategic long-range plan may then be prepared detailing how the mission, in short- and long-range terms, is to be accomplished. Ideally, the mission should be imparted to all management levels; this in turn will trigger the individual objective-setting process.

Objectives should be established on a collective basis with the board and chief executive officer mutually agreeing on specific objectives for each individual. The chief executive officer and chief operating officer will then collectively agree on objectives, and the process will go right down the line with department heads and their immediate supervisors agreeing on objectives.

When first considering an incentive plan, those involved may express concern about the appropriate award criteria. As mentioned, it is not unusual for many executives and even trustees to question whether predetermined, quantifiable targets can be established for the eligible group. Once the discussions begin, however, it becomes apparent that such targets are limited only by the imagination. Invariably the issues to be addressed are not those concerning the identification of incentive targets per se, but rather the identification of those that are directly related to the corporate mission, the long-range plan, or the immediate needs of the organization.

In determining award criteria, the purpose of the plan must be kept in mind—exactly why a system is being contemplated. If the purpose is to reward extraordinary performance, as is usually the case, then such performance levels must be defined. The most pressing concern of the trustees in considering an incentive plan is that individuals not be rewarded for achievements within the scope of their normal job responsibilities. In other words, the threshold of normal performance must be defined. Obviously, this is a difficult task, but it is a critical one. Past performance records and a knowledge of individual capabilities on the part of the chief executive officer are often the determining factors in this area.

Typically, incentive award criteria are frequently expressed in terms of factors such as

- net income as percent of gross revenue;
- cost-per-case reduction;
- daily room-rate reduction;
- cost containment;
- program development and implementation;
- affiliation agreements; and
- market share.

These criteria lend themselves to quantifiable standards. However, this does not and should not preclude the inclusion of more abstract and less quantifiable factors such as quality of care, employee relations, patient relations, and community relations as targets.

As will be seen, the award criteria are frequently the major determining factors in identifying members of the incentive-eligible group. Additional decisions must be made in the identification of incentive targets that consider whether these targets will be expressed in corporate or individual terms or a combination of both.

Specific incentive targets, particularly those of a corporate rather than an individual nature, will probably be imposed on the group.

A question frequently raised by those in the incentive-eligible group concerns the input they will have, if any, regarding the identification of incentive targets. As mentioned, objectives should be established through a collectively and mutually agreed upon process between supervisors and subordinates. Specific incentive targets, particularly those of a corporate rather than an individual nature, will probably be imposed on the group. In the case of an individualized plan, there will be some mutual discussion, but ultimately those objectives that may warrant incentive payment if achieved will be selected by the chief executive officer. In other words, identifying incentive targets may not be a democratic or participatory process.

For those supervisors included in an incentive plan, the award criteria as described will be expressed in terms of specific, predetermined performance and achievement levels beyond the threshold of expected job performance. Objectives, whether corporate or individual, will be defined in highly specific terms with specific completion dates clearly established. The general nebulous objectives common in some elements of health care will no longer be acceptable. These of course are essential elements in any type of management performance appraisal program, but they are especially critical in a performance-based incentive plan.

Eligibility

Eligibility for inclusion in an incentive plan is dependent upon the award criteria. At this time it is most common for eligibility to be restricted to the chief executive officer and his or her immediate subordinates, the rationale being that this is the group most directly responsible for meeting corporate objectives. Even in these situations, however, it is generally the intent of the trustees

and chief executive officer to extend the plan through all management levels if it is successful for the key officer group.

However, much recent evidence suggests that department heads are being included in incentive plans in increasing numbers. This is particularly the case where incentive targets are primarily budgetary. In these instances, department heads with substantial budget responsibility are often included in the incentive-eligible group.

Another factor that must be addressed in determining eligibility for inclusion in an incentive plan consists of the differences in responsibility and in the impact on the organization between line and staff managers. It is not unusual, when the thrust of a plan is on fiscal performance, that only those line managers with direct impact are included. In still other situations, separate nonfiscal incentive targets may be established for staff managers who do not have direct and immediate control in the fiscal area. There are no hard and fast rules, and any manager excluded from participation in an incentive plan may well resent those who are included. However, such potential resentment will not be an overriding factor in determining eligibility. The major consideration will ultimately focus on positions with the most direct and immediate impact on attaining the targets that have been established for incentive purposes.

Invariably the question is raised as to how far down in the organization an incentive plan should be implemented. There is no reason why some type of plan cannot be extended to all levels in the organization. However, the issue may lead to multiple plans, because a plan that is appropriate for the management group will not be appropriate for the rank and file group. There is considerable current discussion in this area, and some hospitals are attempting to establish productivity performance standards for the rank and file that could result in some type of bonus award. Still other institutions are developing pay-for-performance plans for the general employee group to replace the longevity-based, step-rate increase. Such new systems must be carefully defined and designed to ensure virtually complete objectivity in making salary determinations. Ultimately, the most effective approaches for the rank and file employee may be hospitalwide profit sharing or gain sharing plans.

Attitudes

A positive attitude toward the incentive concept on the part of those eligible for participation is absolutely essential if the plan is to succeed. Unlike the business sector in which managers at all levels largely welcome participation in an incentive plan, there is still considerable apprehension toward the concept on the part of many health care managers. This is understandable because of concerns for patient care. More often than not, however, the

concern expressed by health care supervisors centers on the establishment of specific, quantifiable targets. Frankly, being held accountable for meeting specific rather than general objectives has been the exception rather than the rule in not-for-profit health care. This is changing rapidly, however, whether or not incentives are involved.

It is not unusual for concern to be expressed about the creation of a supposedly unhealthy competitive climate within the management group, especially if the targets are individual rather than corporate. A fear often expressed is that the plan will not be fair or equitable. In other words, the belief is fostered that everyone in the incentive-eligible group should be treated alike. However, this is an unreasonable assumption, because the nature of an incentive plan calls for it to identify and reward the high performers.

The broader issue involves ensuring that the plan is administered fairly and in an objective manner. An incentive plan should not be divisive. It should encourage teamwork and cooperation, but the concern for same sometimes reflects the noncompetitive and risk-avoidance nature of many in health care managerial positions. However, health care today requires a willingness to be involved in a competitive endeavor.

If an incentive plan is being considered for an institution, the personnel to be included should ideally be involved in the preliminary discussions. In general, the achievers will be receptive to the idea while the nonachievers will be apprehensive. If one is to be involved in such an undertaking it is critical to assess one's own attitudes, especially if these attitudes are negative. Are you opposed to the concept philosophically, or are you afraid of having your performance measured in definitive terms? Keep an open mind. An incentive system can be a golden opportunity for one's talents and achievements to be recognized.

TYPES OF PLANS

While there are many approaches to incentive system design, most plans fall into two broad categories. The first is the *target,* or *formula,* plan in which awards are based on specific mathematical formulas related to specific achievement levels. The second category is the *discretionary* plan in which awards are not based on specific formulas but are rather subjective. The performance bonus is a typical discretionary plan.

Most of the incentive plans being developed for health care managers are target, or formula, plans. They can be designed to reward group achievement, individual achievement, or both. Incentive funds from which payouts are made can be based on a percentage of net income, savings, aggregate payroll, or an aggregate of the midpoints of the management salary ranges. There are many plans in which each of the incentive targets is assigned a weighting factor. These weightings may be multiplied by base salaries, payroll, or budget targets to ascertain award levels.

Regardless of the type of plan used, however, the most successful are those in which the formulas are easily understood. Participants in a plan should know the formulas and be able to calculate the likely awards based on their progress. Be leery of plans in which the funding and payout formulas are not explained in detail to those in the eligible group and of plans in which the formulas are too mathematically complex.

There are no guarantees of incentive awards. Regardless of group or individual efforts, distribution of the incentive fund is usually predicated upon the institution's net income reaching or exceeding a predetermined level or the institution's controllable costs not exceeding a predetermined level.

Examples of several simple approaches to incentive compensation follow. These are simplified examples and not meant to be definitive by any means.

EFFECT OF A CORPORATE AND INDIVIDUAL INCENTIVE PLAN ON A DEPARTMENT MANAGER EARNING A BASE SALARY OF $35,000 PER YEAR

Conditions

The corporate incentive target is 5 percent net income on gross revenues; the individual incentive target is the reduction of controllable department costs by 5 percent.

The minimum incentive fund is to be 10 percent of eligible payroll; the total payroll of the eligible group is $700,000.

Incentive fund based on corporate target attainment

Actual attained target	Incentive fund as percent of total payroll	
Below 5%		0
5%	10%	$70,000
6%	11%	$77,000
7%	12%	$84,000
8%	13%	$91,000
9%	14%	$98,000
10%	15%	$105,000

The actual corporate target attainment is assumed to be 7 percent of gross revenue.

Potential individual awards are 12 percent of base salary. For a manager earning $35,000 per year, the potential award is $4,200.

The actual individual distribution would be as follows:

Attained individual target	Payout as percent of potential award	
Less than 85% of individual target	0%	0
85–89%	85%	$3,570
90–94%	90%	$3,780
95–99%	95%	$3,990
100–104%	100%	$4,200
105–109%	105%	$4,410
110–114%	110%	$4,620

Another approach is to base award levels on a weighting of the quality of results rather than on specific quantitative levels.

Performance level (incentive targets)	Weighting
Outstanding or superior	100
Excellent	75
Good	50
Unsatisfactory	0
Number in incentive-eligible group	17
Total potential points	1,700

The incentive fund would then be $84,000 (based on 12 percent actual corporate target attainment).

$$\frac{\$84,000}{1,700} = \$49.41 \text{ per point}$$

Award levels:

Less than 50 points		0
	50 points	$2,470
	75 points	$3,705
	100 points	$4,941

RELATIONSHIP OF THE INCENTIVE PLAN TO THE SALARY REVIEW PROCESS

Incentive plans are not designed to replace the annual salary review. They are supplemental forms of compensation that may be awarded for extraordinary performance. It is recognized in most plans that incentive targets may not be reached through no fault of those in the eligible group. Priorities change, and fires have to be put out. Salary reviews should still be based on overall general individual performance and market trends.

There are, however, situations (becoming more common) in which eligibility in an incentive plan may be restricted to those managers whose overall performance ratings are at

Incentive plans are not designed to replace the annual salary review. They are supplemental forms of compensation that may be awarded for extraordinary performance.

least satisfactory if not higher, the assumption being that these are the only managers making a contribution to corporate targets. There are also institutions in which managers whose salary levels are in the upper quartile of their respective salary ranges will be eligible for incentive awards, but additional salary increases will be deferred until such times as there are substantial changes in the market.

CHARACTERISTICS OF VIABLE INCENTIVE PLANS

While there are many approaches to incentive compensation, the most viable plans share the following common characteristics:

- They encourage teamwork and cooperation and are not divisive.
- They are not a substitute for a competitive base salary.
- They are not a "back door" method of granting salary increases.
- Awards are based on specific, not general, achievements.
- Targets are realistic and attainable.
- There are no guarantees of awards.

- Awards are variable and based on the financial condition of the institution.
- Awards are meaningful in terms of effort expended.
- Both group and individual achievements are recognized.
- Long-term as well as short-term achievements are recognized.
- Award formulas are simple and easily understood (this may be the most important criterion).
- Awards are based on quality, not quantity, of result.

• • •

Incentive compensation is rapidly becoming a significant component of health care executive and management compensation programs. While many of the plans involve relatively few people in the top management group, it is only a matter of time before first-line supervisors and department heads are included on a regular basis.

The issues facing health care today dictate that managers now be required to manage in order to ensure the delivery of the highest quality of care in the most efficient, economical manner possible in a highly competitive environment. This will be particularly true of those managers in the professional disciplines who, up to now, have not always recognized or understood their managerial responsibilities, especially concerning the fiscal viability of their employers.

For years, those health care managers who have viewed themselves as the achievers and doers have complained that their achievements and efforts have not been recognized or rewarded. Such efforts and achievements will certainly be recognized in an incentive plan. The risk takers and those unafraid of competition will be and indeed are welcoming the concept with enthusiasm.

Supervisors faced with the pros-pect of being included in an incentive plan should be objective and remain open minded. They should not be afraid to question the plan, however, to ensure that it has been well thought out and is understood by those who are to be included. Most importantly, however, they should view the plan as an opportunity to demonstrate their managerial competence and be rewarded accordingly.

Video display terminals: a new source of employee problems

Charles R. McConnell
Vice President for Employee Affairs
The Genesee Hospital
Rochester, New York

IT IS SAID that those who fail to learn from history are doomed to repeat it. It is also said, somewhat less seriously, that experience is the developed ability to recognize the same mistake twice. That there is more than a trace of truth in these statements is evident in the problems that have arisen around the relative newcomer to the workplace, the video display terminal (VDT).

Also known as the CRT—for cathode ray tube, the television-like tube that provides the screen (although this earlier designation is fading from general use)—the VDT is a major force, if not the single greatest force, in the revolution in office technology. The video display terminal is comparatively new and its use demands major changes in how many employees approach their work.

It has been welcomed by some, approached with caution and suspicion

Health Care Superv, 1985,3(4),81–88
© 1985 Aspen Publishers, Inc.

by others and resisted and resented by many; but for all practical purposes, it is here to stay.

In some respects the video display terminal represents the early 20th century automated assembly line all over again: technology is being developed, introduced and refined far faster than it can be learned, assimilated and accepted. Unlike the case of the assembly line, however, the VDT has sparked concerns for health and safety that have further complicated the problem by polarizing views and solidifying conflicting positions. Labor unions and other interest groups are adopting firm positions on the use of VDTs, positions that sometimes tend to differ widely.

Little scientific evidence has been found of any harmful physical effects from VDTs, although there is much serious study taking place[1]. However, there have been many claims and charges that management has failed to provide a proper work environment for people who work with display terminals.[2]

While the controversy heats up and scientific evidence is as yet inconclusive, it is clear that many employees are having problems. The most frequent employee complaints concerning VDT use involve the eyes—eyestrain, burning, irritation and blurred vision. The next most frequently cited complaints are pain in the back, neck, shoulders and other body members. Also cited often enough to be of genuine concern are increased fatigue, nervousness, and irritability.[3]

GOVERNMENT INVOLVEMENT

A study by the federal Office of Technology Assessment (OTA) suggests that video display terminals pose potential health hazards. The word *potential* must be stressed; study activity notwithstanding, OTA claims that it is still not known whether pregnant women can safely be near terminals all day every workday.[4]

Legislative efforts to regulate the use of video display terminals have been considerably more prominent at the state level than at the federal government level. In California an attempt to mandate alternative work for pregnant VDT operators was voted down in June 1984. The proposed legislation would also have required radiation shielding on all terminals. Business groups lobbied strongly against the bill, legislation which a number of labor unions actively supported. Bills proposing government regulation of VDT use on the job have been introduced in 11 states in addition to California. As of this writing no such bill has become law, but it is possible that one or more may be adopted during 1985.[5]

The most commonly proposed legislation calls for regular vision testing for terminal operators, regular breaks from terminals, a balanced combination of terminal work and nonterminal work and alternative work for pregnant women. A part of several proposed pieces of legislation is a requirement for ergonomically sound work stations; that is, work stations scientifically designed for maximum physical comfort and well being (and thus for maximum efficiency and productivity).

THE UNIONS' POSITION

A number of labor unions are focusing strongly on VDT issues in organizing activities and in contract bargaining. They cite claims of radiation hazards and physical and visual problems resulting from constant terminal use. And since the overwhelming majority of VDT operators are female, the unions also raise the issues of pay inequity, sex discrimination and sex segregation.

Because video display terminals can also be used to monitor operators' work—the terminals are capable of counting keystrokes, recording operating time and otherwise keeping track of output—unions are objecting to having "Big Brother" watching employees as they work. Union representatives claim, perhaps with justification, that electronic work monitoring adds appreciably to job stress.

Some unions are also claiming that the discomfort and stress of terminal work causes VDT operators to experience more illness and absence than employees who do not work at terminals. A study sponsored by The Newspaper Guild, a union with many members who work regularly with VDTs, concluded that on the average terminal users were absent a half-day per year more than nonusers. The Guild study also recommended that federal standards establish breaks

from terminal activity and require regular vision examinations.[6]

The unions have not yet gotten their concerns about VDTs into collective bargaining agreements. However, the United Association of Office, Sales, and Technical Employees did negotiate a side letter to its contract with Wisconsin Electric Power in which the parties agreed to monitor radiation emission levels to ensure employee safety.[7] A scattering of other unions' contracts call for emission monitoring, transfer of pregnant employees and periodic breaks from terminals. Unions are also presenting negotiation demands that call for a mixture of terminal and nonterminal work for employees.

The Communications Workers of America (CWA) has published the CWA Visual Display Terminal Manual, a small book intended to help identify and correct health and safety problems involved in VDT work. Designed as a guide for terminal users, it also specifies what are referred to as standards for terminal installation and operation. The manual discusses possible links of terminal use with birth defects, spontaneous abortion and cataract formation but concedes that no conclusive evidence linking these health hazards to VDTs is available.

THE STATE OF MEDICAL EVIDENCE: INCONCLUSIVE

The Medical Society of New York State opposed proposed VDT legislation in that state, apparently because of lack of hard evidence of radiation hazards. However, this same organization recommended careful attention to workplace design to aid morale and enhance productivity.

In late 1984, tentative evidence that the non-ionizing radiation from VDTs might produce adverse biological effects emerged. However, the evidence was based on experiments that used chick embryos only, and no real link was established between emissions and human health problems.[8] In contrast, the National Institute for Occupational Safety and Health (NIOSH), basing its stand on its research results, does not "see any physiologic mechanism whereby VDTs could impair reproductive function."[9]

At the heart of the discussion of radiation hazard is the contention that VDTs emit low-frequency radiation at levels even less than that of irons, hair dryers and other household appliances. The argument advanced about VDT radiation is the same argument that surrounded color television sets a few years ago.

While industry representatives generally concede some visual and physical effects, as well as the effects of monotony and tension, they take the position that serious radiation hazards do not exist. Industry concedes, however, that all evidence concerning radiation hazards is inconclusive. Organized labor, taking the position that serious radiation hazards do exist, also concedes that the evidence is inconclusive.

It is more than possible that establishment of uniform VDT standards to aid comfortable use by personnel, long a subject of concern to industrial engineers and human factor engineers, may someday find its way into legislation.

A LOOK AT THE WORKPLACE

The radiation controversy has caused some age-old considerations about the physical work area to be overlooked. It is more than possible that establishing uniform work place VDT standards to aid comfortable use by personnel, long a subject of concern to industrial engineers and human factor engineers, may someday find its way into legislation.

Germany has already adopted ergonomic legislation on the premise that preventing long-term orthopedic harm is preferable to paying heavy, continuing compensation claims. In Germany, VDT work surfaces must be 29 inches (72 cm) high, the scientifically established best height for work surfaces used by a sitting worker. Also specified is a minimum work surface width of 48 inches (64 inches is preferred) and a required range of viewing distance (the distance between the operator's eyes and the screen).[10]

Possible legislation notwithstanding, taking a new look at the physical aspects of those office activities that center about video display terminals would seem to make sense. The VDT has vastly increased the physical immobility of office workers and thus has created problems that did not exist before terminals became prevalent. An inch or two of work surface height may make the difference between relative comfort and the aggravation of chronic back pain. The subtleties of lighting may make the difference between visual comfort and eyestrain. The careful placement of a terminal operator's input documents and other necessities may make a difference of thousands of head, neck and eye movements in a workday.

In brief, the VDT workplace must be as carefully engineered as any manufacturing work station where a highly repetitive, physically limiting operation is done.

BACK TO BASICS

In addition to paying careful attention to the ergonomics of the VDT workplace, we need to examine a number of other human factors only lightly touched upon by claims that terminal operators need frequent breaks.

The worker of the 1980s will not readily be assigned to a highly repetitive job that must be done in a relatively fixed position. The worker of 40 to 50 years ago might have settled, uncomplainingly if grudgingly, for a fixed-position assembly line job. He

or she might have become reconciled to working for years at something unpleasant; this was the price one often paid to earn a living. If the work became truly intolerable, the worker would simply quit.

The worker of the 1980s might also quit a job that is repetitive, stressful and limiting. However, the worker of the 1980s is equally as willing—or perhaps even more willing—to challenge the structure and content of the job and try to effect change. Certainly the worker of the 1980s is far more willing to complain openly about job conditions. The complainer of years ago often wound up on the streets seeking new employment. The complainer of today is protected by the law and can usually find someone who is more than willing to listen—social action agencies, local, state and federal government agencies and labor unions. The worker of years ago accepted without question an organization's attitude of: "Here's the job—take it or leave it." Today's worker need not do the same.

A few employees genuinely do not mind highly repetitive work performed in a fixed position. More people, however, prefer some variety in their work; most prefer tasks to be at least somewhat interesting and at least nominally challenging. To a great many workers some degree of autonomy is important, and to many workers some physical mobility is important.

Certainly no single job design or single combination of work procedures, equipment and work space is suitable for everyone. However, as a job becomes routine, repetitive and physically restricting, the number of people who can and will work at that job day in and day out without becoming discontented and unmotivated becomes fewer.

The video display terminal has quickly come to be used for a number of jobs that are routine, repetitive and physically restricting. We have thus come full circle to the early lesson of the automated assembly line: fix a person in one place to one unvarying task, and boredom and monotony soon take their toll. In the case of the VDT, that toll includes physical discomfort, visual discomfort and perhaps tension caused in part by fear of the unknown effects of low-frequency radiation.

Boredom, monotony, immobility, worry about radiation and tension over work monitoring all frequently add up to employee discontent, which inevitably leads to employee relations problems, which in turn lead to reduced productivity.

There is of course a certain engineering logic behind the division of labor of early factory automation and current manufacturing operations. Grouping tasks certainly improves efficiency and increases output. The worker who performs the same group of well-defined motions over and over again invariably turns out more quantity than the worker who performs dissimilar tasks.

VDT technology has been largely responsible for the intrusion of the manufacturing division of labor concept into the office environment. For example, a secretary, typist or billing clerk in pre–VDT days had a modest amount of mobility and a variety of tasks to perform. The VDT, however, will not do everything these people have done, and VDTs cost too much to be provided to each worker. Division of labor places similar tasks together; in the case of the VDT, similar tasks are all keyboard tasks. Thus some of the work of the secretary, some of the work of the typist and some of the work of the billing clerk become the work of one person assigned to one VDT, creating restrictive combinations of similar work as surely as did Henry Ford's first automobile manufacturing operation.

The experience of the last several decades suggests that the price of productive efficiency is often far too high in terms of the human problems that result from placing people in rigidly engineered working situations. This is supposedly an era of enlightenment in management, a time marked by a steady shift toward people-centered management. Yet the narrower the division of labor becomes in search of productive efficiency, the greater is the pull back toward production-centered management—management that focuses primarily on process and output, and secondarily or perhaps only incidentally on the worker. The further a job and worker go toward production-centered management, the greater is the likelihood of employee discontent.

Much like the photocopiers that in the not-too-distant past caused something of a revolution in office practices, VDTs are here to stay—at least until their functions can be performed better, faster and more economically by some yet-to-be-developed technology.

It is therefore necessary for supervisors and employees to learn to live with VDTs, viewing them as tools to help people get their work done, and remembering that people, not machinery, control the work pace and accomplishment tasks.

Bringing in the VDT as a tool for people may mean sacrificing some of the productive efficiency that strict division of labor provides. It may mean rearranging tasks to create jobs that are not exclusively terminal-operator positions but that are combinations of terminal assignments and other tasks. Truly enlightened management should not have to be forced by legislation to require periodic breaks from terminal work or to balance terminal with nonterminal work. Enlightened management, putting person before process in job design, should render much proposed VDT legislation unnecessary.

A final word in this discussion of video display terminals is more appropriately directed at terminal-using workers rather than their supervisors. Much of the negative reaction to VDTs has risen from simple resistance to change.

In years past the introduction of another technological innovation also created much consternation. This innovation was accused of bringing hazards into the work place and was condemned as representing unnecessary displacement of the old way of doing things. A few welcomed the new technology with open arms; some silently but grudgingly came around after a while; more than just a few resisted and went to extremes to retain the old way. As a result this particular new technology required much more time to achieve general acceptance than its proponents had predicted. This technological innovation that upset so many people was the electric typewriter.

REFERENCES

1. Research Institute of America. *Employment Alert*, "Office Administration and Work Place Stress Examined in Congressional Report." (October 18, 1984): 5.
2. "Failure to Provide Proper Work Environment Real Source of Ills." *Infosystems* 31, no. 10 (1984): 17.
3. Ibid.
4. Bureau of National Affairs. "Potential Hazards to Office Workers Cited in OTA Study." *White Collar Report* 56 (September 19, 1984): 339.
5. Bureau of National Affairs. "Tom Hayden's VDT Bill Bites Dust in California Assembly Vote." *White Collar Report* 56 (July 11, 1984): 41.
6. American Society for Personnel Administration. "VDT Users Sick More Often Than Nonusers." *Resource* (January 1984): 12.
7. Bureau of National Affairs. "Wisconsin Utility Agrees to Monitor VDTs in Settlement with Independent Union." *White Collar Report* 55 (April 4, 1984): 400.

8. Bureau of National Affairs. "New VDT Radiation Research Said to Produce Adverse Biological Effects." *White Collar Report* 56 (October 24, 1984): 509.

9. Bureau of National Affairs. "No VDT Reproductive Risk Seen, But NIOSH Study Planned, Hill Panel Told." *White Collar Report* 55 (May 16, 1984): 577.

10. Wehr, W. "Europe Is Living (And Working) with New Furniture Standards." *Modern Office Technology* 29, no. 5 (1984): 132.

Improving productivity in the health care industry: An argument and supporting evidence from one hospital

Michael Koshuta
Assistant Professor of Management
Purdue University—North Central
Westville, Indiana

Michael K. McCuddy
Professor of Human Resource Management
College of Business Administration
Valparaiso University
Valparaiso, Indiana

OBSERVERS OF THE health care industry in the United States have sounded an ominous alarm. A typical prediction follows:

The health care environment of tomorrow will be more hostile and competitive than today. The hospital industry is in transition. By the year 2000, market failure and takeover of some hospitals is likely. Third party insurers and government will refuse to provide a safety net for overpriced and mismanaged hospitals.[1]

The health care industry must become less concerned about getting more money from third party insurers and government to cover its inefficiencies. Instead, the industry must become more concerned about reducing costs within its own controllable arena so it can survive with the funds that will be avail-

An earlier version of a portion of this article was presented at the National Meeting of the Academy of Management in Anaheim, California on August 7–10, 1988.

Health Care Superv 1989, 8(1), 15-30

able. The health care industry must learn how to live within its means while assuring the public that the quality and quantity of its services will be maintained.

Gray and Steffy provide a response to the problem of cost control.

As pressures increase on hospital managers to reduce the rate of operating cost increases, the need to examine management philosophies and practices becomes necessary. Old cost reimbursement orientations must be replaced with a focus on, and daily attention to, cost containment, productivity monitoring, and sound business planning. Although some hospital executives have found that, during the transition to a more rational and less regulated health delivery system, cost containment has actually resulted in lower operating margins, nevertheless it is only a matter of time until the hospital will have to be managed like any other business operating in a competitive environment. The hospital must become a financially sound enterprise, rather than a funded operation.[2]

OVERVIEW OF THE PRODUCTIVITY IMPROVEMENT PROGRAM

The productivity improvement program consisted of four separate but integrated components for improving hospital productivity. One component was the development of a team-oriented work system to facilitate and enhance the hospital staff's willingness and ability to work together effectively to improve productivity. A second component was the development of a system for measuring and monitoring productivity. A third component involved the setting of goals for improving productivity (or, in the case of departments that were already highly productive, maintaining productivity). A fourth component was the development of a team-oriented reward system to reinforce the hospital's staff in attaining their productivity goals. In short, the entire productivity improvement program consisted of developing and using a team-oriented work system to achieve measurable productivity goals and then reinforcing the attainment of those productivity goals through the use of a team-oriented reward system.

TEAM-ORIENTED WORK SYSTEM

Work systems integrate many different variables, including but not limited to the way jobs are designed; the nature of supervision; the nature and extent of employee participation, if any, in the organization's goal-setting and decision-making processes; and the relative emphasis on individualism versus teamwork.[3] While Beer and colleagues[4] discuss two opposing work systems, it is suggested here that work systems may be conceptualized on a continuum. One extreme of the continuum would be represented by highly specialized and extremely routine jobs, very close and highly directive supervision, no employee participation, and an individualistic orientation. The opposite end of the continuum would be characterized by broadly defined and complex jobs, self- or peer-supervision, broad employee participation, and an extremely heavy reliance on teamwork. Various types of team-oriented work systems would exist on the upper portion of the continuum.

Because of the interdependent nature of much of the hospital's activities, it may be argued that some form of team-oriented work system would facilitate attempts to improve productivity.

Organizational survey

It was necessary to assess the nature of the existing work system at the hospital studied. A survey measuring various aspects of the work system was distributed to all members of the hospital's staff excluding the physicians and surgeons holding staff privileges. Of 525 nonsupervisory personnel employed at the time of survey distribution, 444 (84.6%) completed the form. Nearly all the managerial and supervisory personnel completed the survey (74 of 80 or 92.5%).

Through a series of structured questions, the survey form assessed nine aspects of the system:

1. The motivating potential of employees' jobs.
2. The supervisors' and work group members' emphasis on developing positive working relationships.
3. The supervisors' and work group members' support for work activities.
4. The supervisors' and work group members' commitment to goal attainment and excellence.
5. The supervisors' and work group members' emphasis on employee growth and development.
6. The supervisors' and work group members' commitment to teamwork.
7. The working relationships between the employees' department and other departments in the hospital.
8. The importance of job context factors (e.g., fair treatment from supervisors, compensation, fringe benefits, and relationships with coworkers).
9. The importance of job content factors (e.g., stimulating, challenging, and responsible work; growth and learning opportunities; and accomplishment on the job).

From a diagnostic perspective, it may be argued that items 1 through 7 measure what the hospital's existing work system provides in terms of a team-oriented system, and item 9 measures the employees' potential or desire to respond to a team-oriented work system. Several parts of the structured portion of the survey were adapted from Hackman and Oldham, Dyer, and several surveys that had been used in other organizations, including hospitals.[5,6] Additional questions were designed based on the findings of a pilot study in two of the hospital's departments (radiology and environmental services). It should be noted that a detailed description of the psychometric properties of the various measurement scales on the survey forms is beyond the scope and purpose of this article, but such information is available from the authors on request.

In addition to the structured questions, the survey contained several essay questions. One question asked employees to indicate what type of reward they wanted in return for improved productivity. Additional essay questions concerned the employees' perceptions of their department's main strengths and weaknesses regarding efforts to improve productivity and ways productivity might be improved within and between departments.

Survey feedback and team development within departments

Information from the organizational survey was given to the supervisory and nonsupervisory personnel in each department. The survey data consisted of hospitalwide averages and departmental averages on the structured diagnostic variables and a summary of employees' responses to the essay questions. After the survey results were provided, team development proceeded by having each department identify the areas it wished to work on in terms of improving the way department members worked together. Action plans were then developed and implemented.

In several of the departments, particularly in the nursing units, the survey feedback provided the impetus for personnel to finally confront problems they knew existed but had avoided solving. The survey feedback was, in a sense, cathartic; the problems were finally out in the open, and people were relieved. Discussion of the problems generated commitment to change as well as realistic and meaningful action plans for implementing changes.

Many of the action plans concerned how people would deal with each other in terms of solving problems and resolving conflicts, as well as how they could help each other and work together more effectively. These action plans have been implemented by the various departments with varying degrees of success. In most cases, however, personnel in the various departments now recognize that they are members of a team that must function effectively if the department is to make a meaningful contribution to both quality patient care and productivity.

Interdepartmental team development

Because of the interdependent nature of many of the hospital's activities and because some of the productivity gains would need to be realized across departments, it was

Specific activities were undertaken to develop the capabilities of each interdepartmental team to function effectively in a team-oriented environment.

necessary to establish a mechanism for solving problems and conflicts that existed between departments and could affect productivity. This mechanism took the form of interdepartmental teams of various department directors. These teams were formed initially on the basis of how critical other departments were to the effective operation of one's own department.

Initial membership of the interdepartmental teams cut across normal reporting lines. Over time, however, and with some restructuring of organizational reporting relationships, the membership on the interdepartmental teams became identical to normal lines of authority. One team, for example, initially consisted of directors from admitting, medical care evaluation, medical records, social services, patient accounting, data processing, and home health care. All but the last three departments reported to one upper-level manager. Patient accounting and data processing reported to a different manager and home health care did not have a direct reporting relationship to any higher-level manager. After much work, the medical management team now consists of admitting, medical care evaluation, medical records, social services, patient accounting, and home health care. Furthermore, all these departments now report to the same upper-level manager.

Specific activities were undertaken to develop the capabilities of each interdepartmental team to function effectively in a team-oriented environment. Initially, each team decided which interdepartmental problems it would attempt to address. Subsequently, each interdepartmental team met periodically to explore new problems and to review progress on solving previously identified problems. As a result of these periodic efforts, a more cooperative working relationship has emerged among the various departments.

PRODUCTIVITY MEASUREMENT SYSTEM

The productivity measurement system was developed using three guiding principles. The first principle was a conceptual model of productivity. This model viewed productivity as a function of three variables—output, input, and quality—as shown in equation 1.

$$\text{Productivity} = \frac{\text{output}}{\text{input}} \; x \; \text{quality} \quad (1)$$

The second principle was that the productivity measurement system had to be inexpensive, in terms of both development and administration. Therefore, where possible, existing data were used as a basis for determining the productivity standards for each department. The third principle was that the department directors should participate in the development of their department's productivity measurement system and should be willing to commit their department to being measured and evaluated under that system.

In many departments, output was measured by using revenue generated by the department and input was measured by using cost incurred by the department. Table 1 indicates which departments followed the revenue and cost approach. In those departments that were not adaptable to use of a revenue-to-cost ratio, different methods of measuring output and input were devised. The particular method of measurement varied from department to department, as shown in Table 1. In one instance (guild/volunteers), only output could be identified or meaningfully measured. In three cases (telephone and information, safety/security, and boiler), a quality measure was used as the sole component of productivity measurement. On balance, however, most departments followed the output–input conceptualization set forth in equation 1.

The measurement of quality basically is conceptualized as a percentage adjustment to the output–input ratio. When work is performed without flaw (100% quality), the productivity index is equal to the output–input ratio. When quality is less than 100%, the productivity index is less than the output–input ratio.

Unfortunately, the quality component of the productivity index has not been fully developed and implemented in all departments. In those departments where it has been developed and implemented (medical management, telephone and information, safety/security, and boiler), the actual quality figures have been incorporated into each department's productivity index. In all the departments where the quality measurement is still under development, quality was assumed to be 100% in the respective productivity indices.

It should be noted that the method for deriving this percentage adjustment for quality will differ among the various depart-

Table 1. Output and input used in departmental productivity measurement systems

Hospital department	Output	Input
Diagnostic services team		
Cardiac services	Revenue	Cost
Pharmacy	Revenue	Cost
Laboratory/blood bank	Revenue	Cost
Occupational/physical therapy	Revenue	Cost
Respiratory therapy	Revenue	Cost
Nuclear medicine	Revenue	Cost
Combined radiologic services	Revenue	Cost
Medical management team		
Medical management department[*]	Bills processed	Paid hours
Guild/volunteers	Hours of volunteer service provided to hospital	
Telephone and information[†]		
Home health care	Revenue	Cost
Nursing team		
Intensive care unit	Acuity hours	Actual hours
Telemetry unit	Acuity hours	Actual hours
Medical/surgical (unit 1)	Acuity hours	Actual hours
Obstetrics/nursery	Acuity hours	Actual hours
Pediatrics	Acuity hours	Actual hours
Rehabilitation	Acuity hours	Actual hours
Medical/surgical (unit 2)	Acuity hours	Actual hours
Medical/surgical (unit 3)	Acuity hours	Actual hours
Surgery/ambulatory services/emergency team		
Surgery/recovery	Revenue	Cost
Ambulatory services	Revenue	Cost
Emergency department	Revenue	Cost
Support services team		
Combined supply, purchasing, and distribution	Revenue	Cost
Safety/security[†]		
Environmental services	Standard hours	Actual hours
Dietary	Revenue	Cost
Engineering services	Standard hours	Actual hours
Boiler[‡]		
Laundry	Utilization	Capacity
Administrative team		
General accounting	Achievement	Goals
Electronic data processing	Achievement	Goals
Community relations	Achievement	Goals
Administrative (clerical)	Achievement	Goals
Pastoral care	Achievement	Goals
Personnel	Achievement	Goals

[*] The medical management department is a "super department" because it consists of a number of others, in this case, admitting, patient accounting, medical records, social service, and utilization review/quality assurance.

[†] The productivity index for telephone and information and safety/security is entirely a quality measure. Each legitimate complaint about service provided results in a 5% reduction of the productivity index. Thus, 100% indicates that perfect service was rendered during the measurement period, while 95% signifies that one legitimate complaint about service was received during the measurement period.

[‡] The productivity index for the boiler is a quality measure predicated on the continuous availability of steam pressure with a minimum acceptable response time to correct pressure deviations. Each response that exceeds the minimum response time is subject to a 5% deduction in the productivity index. Thus, 100% indicates that all responses to pressure deviations are at or below minimum.

ments. For example, in the laboratory and blood bank the quality factor will be measured as shown in equation 2.

$$\text{Quality} = 1 - \frac{\substack{\text{number of physician} \\ \text{complaints regarding} \\ \text{incorrect tests}}}{\substack{\text{total number of} \\ \text{tests performed}}} \quad (2)$$

In the medical management department quality is measured by equation 3.

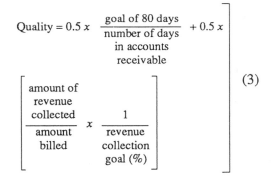

$$\text{Quality} = 0.5 \, x \left[\frac{\text{goal of 80 days}}{\substack{\text{number of days} \\ \text{in accounts} \\ \text{receivable}}} + 0.5 \, x \right.$$

$$\left. \left[\frac{\substack{\text{amount of} \\ \text{revenue} \\ \text{collected}}}{\substack{\text{amount} \\ \text{billed}}} \, x \, \frac{1}{\substack{\text{revenue} \\ \text{collection} \\ \text{goal (\%)}}} \right] \right] \quad (3)$$

In the nursing units, quality will be measured with a demerit system wherein percentage deductions in quality are made based on the severity of verified and justified complaints (e.g., a lost lawsuit would automatically reduce the quality factor to zero and negate any productivity improvement; not responding to a patient's call within a specified period of time, considering census, would result in a deduction of 2.5%. This quality measure has not yet been incorporated into the nursing departments' productivity index because the system for collecting the data is still being developed.

A final comment should be made regarding the productivity measurement system. The authors sought to generate data for the productivity indices beginning with the first quarter of 1985. However, because of the variety of ways in which output, input, and quality are operationalized in order for each department's productivity index to be meaningful, data are not consistently available across this period.

The quarterly data reflect three distinct periods for the entire productivity improvement program: (1) the period before the introduction of the productivity improvement program, consisting of six quarters, from the first quarter of 1985 through the second quarter of 1986; (2) the period during the design and implementation of the productivity improvement program, encompassing the third and fourth quarters of 1986; and (3) the period after implementation of the productivity improvement program, reflecting the four quarters of 1987.

SETTING PRODUCTIVITY GOALS

The productivity measurement system provided the basis for each department to set a goal for improving productivity during 1987. The goal-setting process differed among the departments depending on the presence or absence of baseline productivity indices and whether the productivity measurement system itself was adaptable to a management by objectives (MBO) process.

Departments with baseline productivity indices

In all the departments where baseline productivity indices were present, the following procedure was used for setting productivity goals. First, standard work-sampling methods from industrial engineering were applied to monthly productivity data from the baseline period so a beginning productivity standard could be derived for the department.[7] This beginning productivity standard was basically the average of the top quartile of the department's monthly productivity figures (excluding justifiable outliers). The consultants then reviewed the beginning productivity standard with the department's director and upper management. If this review indicated that the department was operating at less than an optimum level during the selected months, a productivity improvement goal was established.

Productivity improvement goals were set anywhere from 5% to 15%, depending on the department. For example, if a department's beginning productivity standard was 3.17 and the goal was to improve productivity by 5%, the beginning standard was given an efficiency rating of 95% ($1 - .05 = .95$), resulting in the final productivity standard of 3.34 ($3.34 = 3.17/.95$). This final productivity standard of 3.34 implicitly recognized 100% quality and was the productivity index the department in the example had to meet to achieve its productivity improvement goal. It should be noted that this illustrative department could have met the final productivity standard by having an output–input ratio of 3.34 and maintaining quality at 100%, or by having an output–input ratio in excess of 3.34 while allowing quality to drop below 100%.

If the review of the beginning productivity standard revealed that the department was operating at optimum level during the selected months, the goal became one of maintaining productivity rather than improving productivity. In such a case, the beginning standard became the final productivity standard.

During the post-intervention period, the extent of productivity goal attainment was assessed on a quarterly basis. For each department, a quarterly average of the three monthly productivity figures was computed and then compared with the final productivity standard. If the quarterly average met or exceeded the standard, the department had realized its productivity goal during the quarter. If the quarterly average fell short of the final productivity standard, the department had failed to achieve its productivity goal.

Departments without baseline productivity indices

A somewhat different goal-setting procedure was used in those departments where productivity information was not available before or during the intervention period but was available after the intervention period. In those departments, productivity improvement goals were set on the basis of the collective judgment of the department director, upper management, and consultants regarding what the productivity index should be if the department performed well. This figure represented the final productivity standard. The evaluation of goal attainment was conducted in the same manner as described above.

Departments exclusively adaptable to the MBO process

For the departments of the administrative team, where no historical data were applicable, productivity was determined through a management by objectives (MBO) process that specifically set goals, priorities, and time and cost constraints for each quarter. In setting goals and evaluating the extent of goal attainment, the directors of each department on the administrative team reviewed each other's goals prior to the goals being reviewed by the hospital's chief administrator. This two-level review ensured the integrity of the process.

If the goals set through the MBO process were achieved, the department was considered to have realized its quarterly productivity goal. If these goals were not achieved, the department did not meet its quarterly productivity goal.

TEAM-ORIENTED REWARD SYSTEM

One question on the organizational survey asked employees to indicate the type of reward they would like in return for increased productivity. The most frequently identified reward by both nonsupervisory personnel and managerial or supervisory personnel was money. Since money was the most desired reward and since a team-oriented work system was being used because of the highly interdependent nature of much of the hospital's work, it was decided to develop a gain-sharing reward system.[8]

The reward for achieving the productivity goals is a share in the quarterly profits generated by the hospital. For a gain-sharing reward distribution to occur, the hospital must make a profit during the measurement period. If a profit is made, part of the profit goes to the hospital and the remainder goes to the employee gain-sharing distribution pool. This distribution pool is divided into three parts: the hospital pool shared by all employees, the team pool shared by all members of the interdepartmental teams that meet or exceed their team goal, and the departmental pool shared by those departments that meet or exceed their department's productivity goal. For example, if there is a profit and a specific interdepartmental team achieves the team productivity goal (e.g., the average percent of goal attainment for all departments on the team must equal or exceed 100%) but one department on the team does not achieve its departmental productivity goal, that department would participate in the hospital and team pools but not in the departmental pool. Assuming, however, that all the other departments on this interdepartmental team achieved their departmental productivity goal, each of the remaining departments would share in the hospital, team, and departmental pools.

PRODUCTIVITY IMPROVEMENT RESULTS

Longitudinal comparisons of productivity indices

Longitudinal comparisons are not provided for the nursing team and the administrative team since productivity data are available for both teams only during the four quarters of 1987. However, longitudinal comparisons are provided for the diagnostic services team, the medical management team, the surgery/ambulatory services/ emergency team, and the support services team, since productivity data are available before, during, and after the productivity improvement intervention.

To track productivity improvement over time, a productivity improvement factor for each department was calculated by dividing the productivity index for the first available quarter into the productivity index for subsequent quarters. The productivity improvement factors were then analyzed in two ways: with the t test for correlated data and with graphs.[9]

Table 2 provides the results of t tests performed on comparisons of productivity improvement factors before, during, and

Table 2. Results of t tests on productivity improvement factors using methodology for correlated data

Hospital unit	During vs. before intervention	After vs. during intervention	After vs. before intervention
Diagnostic services team			
Average	0.1303	0.1905	0.3208
Variance	0.0077	0.0077	0.0072
Sample size	7.0000	7.0000	7.0000
t value	3.9265[*]	5.7602[†]	9.9796[†]
Medical management team[‡]			
Average	0.2465	0.0316	0.2781
Variance	0.0319	0.0020	0.0301
Sample Size	3.0000	3.0000	3.0000
t value	2.3889[§]	1.2329	2.7749[§]
Surgery/ambulatory service/emergency team			
Average	0.0703	0.2531	0.3235
Variance	0.0107	0.0512	0.0151
Sample size	3.0000	3.0000	3.0000
t value	1.1769	1.9377[§]	4.5552[¶]
Support services team[‖]			
Average	0.0161	0.0290	0.0451
Variance	0.0011	0.0015	0.0012
Sample size	5.0000	5.0000	5.0000
t value	1.0956	1.6729	2.8735[¶]

[*] $p < .005$.
[†] $p < .001$.
[‡] Excludes telephone and information department since data were not available for this unit before, during, and after the intervention period.
[§] $p < .10$.
[¶] $p < .05$.
[‖] Excludes environmental services and engineering services departments since data were not available for these units before, during, and after the intervention period.

after the intervention period. Comparison of productivity improvement factors before and after the intervention clearly demonstrates that the productivity improvement program significantly increased productivity in each of the four interdepartmental teams identified in Table 2. Moreover, the activities in the two quarters during which the intervention was designed and implemented also significantly improved productivity on the diagnostic services team and the medical management team.

Further insight into the longitudinal data can be gained by examining the graphic presentations of the quarterly data. On the diagnostic services team, the surgery/ambulatory services/emergency team, and the medical management team, a general trend of productivity improvement occurred over the six quarters preceding the intervention period (see Figure 1). However, during the intervention period, productivity improvement declined on the diagnostic services team and surgery/ambulatory services/emergency team but continued to increase on the medical management team.

The decline on the diagnostic services team and surgery/ambulatory services/emergency team was probably because (1) considerable administrative time was spent "selling" the productivity measurement and teamwork concepts to the departments on the respective teams; (2) considerable administrative time was spent assisting in the development of the productivity measurement system; and (3) considerable time was spent by department directors and nonsupervisory personnel in necessary teambuilding activities. However, the time was a worthwhile investment, as evidenced by the sharp increases in these two team's productivity improvement factors after the intervention period (see Figure 1).

The continued productivity improvement during the intervention period for the medical management team may have been due, in part, to the consultants serving as an effective buffer between team members who were having significant interpersonal problems. Once the consultants exited the hospital at the end of 1986 and no longer served as buffers, the interpersonal problems reemerged and interfered with efforts to function as a work team. These interpersonal difficulties were eventually resolved, however, and teamwork again improved. This interpretation is supported by the upward trend in the productivity improvement factor after the intervention period (see Figure 1).

The productivity improvement factor did not show a pronounced trend for the support services team before the intervention period; instead it bounced around quite a bit. During the intervention period there was a decline, which can probably be explained by the reasons already cited above. After the intervention period, productivity rose and remained fairly stable.

The productivity improvement program contributed to significant and substantial gains in productivity for all the interdepartmental teams.

Overall, the longitudinal data clearly and strongly indicate that the productivity improvement program contributed to significant and substantial gains in productivity for all the interdepartmental teams for which data were available before, during, and after the intervention.

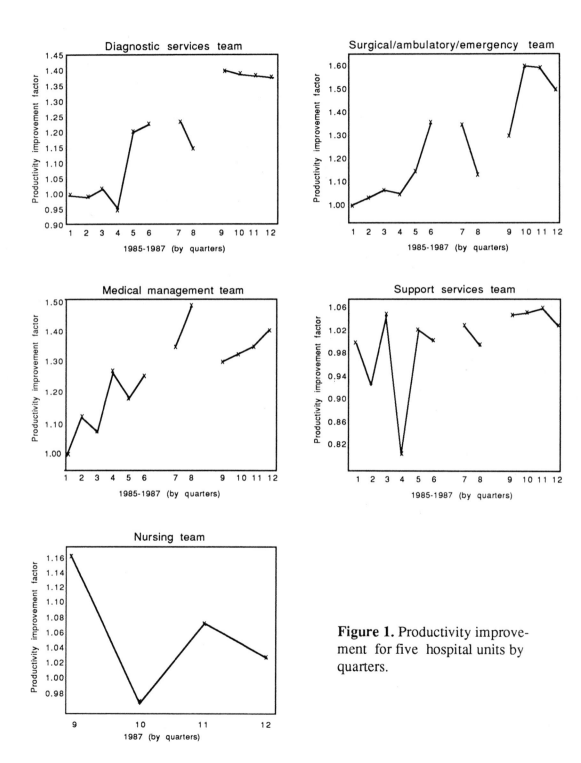

Figure 1. Productivity improvement for five hospital units by quarters.

Attainment of productivity goals

As mentioned earlier, each hospital department established a productivity goal for 1987. Actual productivity results were then compared with the productivity goals to determine the extent of goal attainment.

For the departments on the diagnostic services team, the medical management team, the surgery/ambulatory services/emergency team, and the support services team, a percentage of goal attainment was calculated by dividing the productivity goal into the actual productivity results. The productivity goal attainment figures for the above teams and the nursing team are presented in Table 3. Overall, three of the above teams exceeded their productivity goals by slightly more than 3%, while the fourth team exceeded its goal by more than 8%. This achievement is particularly impressive given that the productivity goals were established at levels 5% to 15% above the top quartile of the baseline productivity figures. Thus, the total difference between 1986 and 1987 actually reflects productivity gains in excess of the 3% to 8% that was realized on goal attainment.

The nursing team's productivity improvement factor reflects the ratio of nursing hours per patient day required by patient acuity to actual nursing hours used per patient day. The nursing team departments' productivity goal is realized when the productivity improvement factor (the ratio of required nursing hours to actual nursing hours) is 1.0, thereby signifying a perfect match between the nursing care required by patient acuity and the nursing care provided. A productivity improvement factor of less than 1.0 reflects some degree of over-staffing, and an improvement factor greater

than 1.0 indicates some degree of under-staffing. The productivity improvement factors for the nursing team in Table 3 show a definite trend toward more optimal staffing (e.g., an improvement factor of 1.0) over the four quarters of 1987 (see Figure 1).

However, the nursing team figures can be a bit misleading for three reasons. First, there is a learning curve effect, since the nursing team departments only began using the acuity system in the first quarter of 1987. Second, the acuity system does not account for patients who are on holding status (e.g., patients not officially admitted to a department but whose care is the responsibility of that department). Third, the acuity system does not adequately account for variations in the mix of nursing personnel (registered nurses, licensed practical nurses, and nurse's aides) that are available to the nursing team departments. Yet different personnel mixes influence the number of nursing hours that are actually used as well as the quality of care that can be provided to patients. (Incidentally, in an effort to address the latter two problems, appropriate refinements of the acuity measurement system are being considered.)

The administrative team's productivity goal attainment was entirely a function of whether the departments achieved the goals set through the MBO process. Data show that every administrative team department met its productivity goal in every quarter.

Cost savings realized from exceeding productivity goals

Cost savings realized during 1987 because of productivity goal attainment were calculated for departments that used reve-

Table 3. 1987 productivity improvement results relative to 1987 productivity improvement goal

Diagnostic services team (Hospital department)	Percent of productivity goal attainment				
	Q1	Q2	Q3	Q4	Average
Cardiac services	126.74	115.12	116.36	117.60	118.95
Pharmacy	106.88	105.88	108.03	105.78	106.64
Laboratory/blood bank	101.66	98.27	101.49	117.64	104.87
Occupational/physical therapy	95.86	99.17	116.29	111.63	105.74
Respiratory therapy	103.49	88.13	91.76	85.66	92.26
Nuclear medicine	100.01	108.50	89.74	73.13	92.85
Combined radiologic services	99.92	113.05	100.34	104.92	104.68
Team average	104.94	104.02	103.43	102.34	103.68

Medical management team (Hospital department)	Percent of productivity goal attainment				
	Q1	Q2	Q3	Q4	Average
Medical management department	102.56	117.95	112.82	112.82	111.54
Guild/volunteers	87.85	101.46	98.59	118.61	101.63
Telephone and information	90.00	95.00	100.00	100.00	96.25
Home health care	110.97	96.01	104.74	103.87	103.90
Team average	97.85	102.60	104.04	108.82	103.33

Surgery/ambulatory services/emergency team (Hospital department)	Percent of productivity goal attainment				
	Q1	Q2	Q3	Q4	Average
Surgery/recovery	98.02	101.40	104.99	94.96	99.84
Ambulatory services	99.95	156.17	127.11	131.30	128.63
Emergency department	84.70	87.46	113.33	99.02	96.13
Team average	94.23	115.01	115.14	108.43	108.20

Support services team (Hospital department)	Percent of productivity goal attainment				
	Q1	Q2	Q3	Q4	Average
Combined supply, purchasing, and distribution	117.47	115.57	117.86	99.39	112.57
Safety/security	100.00	100.00	95.00	100.00	98.75
Environmental services	95.00	97.50	98.75	96.25	96.88
Dietary	100.71	95.73	101.83	105.69	100.99
Engineering services	106.61	98.65	102.40	91.59	99.81
Boiler	109.22	107.44	111.11	109.22	109.25
Laundry	91.38	110.68	105.53	105.53	103.28
Team average	102.91	103.65	104.64	101.10	103.08

Nursing team (Hospital department)	1987				
	Q1	Q2	Q3	Q4	Average
Intensive care unit	1.1769*	1.1538	1.0373	1.0075	1.0939
Telemetry unit	1.4182	1.1455	1.0741	1.0000	1.1594
Medical/surgical (unit 1)	0.8852	0.8197	1.1136	1.0192	0.9594
Obstetrics/nursery	1.6071	0.7857	1.0833	1.0556	1.1329
Pediatrics	1.2344	1.0156	1.0000	0.9649	1.0537
Rehabilitation	0.8214	1.0000	1.0862	1.1034	1.0028
Medical/surgical (unit 2)	1.0926	0.9259	1.1111	1.0385	1.0420
Medical/surgical (unit 3)	1.0385	0.9615	1.0638	1.0600	1.0310
Team average	1.1593	0.9760	1.0712	1.0311	1.0594

*Productivity improvement factor = Acuity hours/actual hours.

nue and expense for the output–input ratio or that used labor hours as the input measure (see Table 4). Cost savings were computed with the following formulas:

$$\begin{matrix} \text{Cost} \\ \text{savings} \end{matrix} = \begin{matrix} \text{cost at 100\%} \\ \text{efficiency} \end{matrix} - \begin{matrix} \text{cost actually} \\ \text{incurred in 1987} \end{matrix} \quad (4)$$

where

$$\begin{matrix} \text{Cost at 100\%} \\ \text{efficiency} \end{matrix} = \frac{\text{1987 revenues}}{\text{1987 productivity goal}} \quad (5)$$

The total cost savings realized by the departments mentioned was $681,328. In different terms, if the departments' productivity improvement goals had been met but not exceeded, costs of $11,660,988 would have been incurred. By collectively exceeding the productivity improvement goals, the departments incurred only $10,979,660.

•   •   •

The productivity improvement program described in this article has produced significant and substantial results for one hospital. Productivity goals have been achieved, and substantial cost savings have been realized. In short, this hospital has responded in the manner advocated at the outset of this article. But this hospital still is not out of the woods in terms of dealing effectively with its competitive environment. It must continue working to improve productivity to the optimum level and to maintain it once the optimum level is reached. To do otherwise is to court failure in an increasingly hostile and competitive environment.

The hospital is still in a tough position for several reasons. First, while some departments have done very well, others need to

Table 4. Cost savings realized by departments

Hospital department	Cost savings ($)
Diagnostic services team	
Cardiac services	74,049
Pharmacy	79,038
Laboratory/blood bank	73,269
Occupational/physical therapy	6,506
Respiratory therapy	-28,275
Nuclear medicine	-15,187
Combined radiologic services	32,838
Team total	222,237
Medical management team	
Medical management department*	150,130
Home health care	13,967
Team total	164,097
Surgery ambulatory services/emergency team	
Surgery/recovery	-4,772
Ambulatory services	68,965
Emergency department	-13,595
Team total	50,598
Support services team	
Combined supply, purchasing, and distribution	208,466
Environmental services*	-23,028
Dietary	59,880
Engineering services*	922
Team total	244,396
Grand total	681,328

*Based on hours saved.

work much more vigorously at productivity improvement. This problem occurs whenever a team orientation is applied to complex organization; some departments may not carry their weight.

Second, in the past this hospital's personnel often did not think or behave in terms of functioning in a team environment. With the productivity improvement program, they were required to develop new ways of working together effectively. However, these methods have not yet been fully developed, and personnel must continue to work on them.

Third, in this hospital (and probably throughout the health care industry), managerial and supervisory personnel such as patient care directors (head nurses), laboratory directors, surgery and recovery room supervisors, and radiology department heads traditionally have viewed themselves as clinicians supervising the delivery of quality patient care. Now these managers must be clinical managers as well as business managers, roles they may view as conflicting.

Fourth, the hospital's personnel must come to grips with an increasingly prevalent feature of the competitive environment, that the ability to continue providing quality health care is based on being productive, containing costs, and using resources wisely. These requirements necessitate a significant shift in thinking for many employees at this hospital (and throughout the health care industry). People must change the ingrained ideology that hospitals are not factories and therefore should not be subjected to a productivity philosophy. A new philosophy is needed if hospitals are to survive and continue to provide quality health care to as many people as possible at a reasonable cost.

In short, this hospital's problems are associated with a multipronged attempt to alter the organization's culture. Without these cultural changes, productivity improvements may not be sustained over the long term and the productivity philosophy may not become an ongoing, integral part of how this hospital conducts its business affairs.

Based on the experience thus far with one hospital, the authors believe that the four-part productivity improvement program holds substantial promise for application to other hospitals in the United States. If implemented and used continuously and properly, it will provide a means of effective management and competition for any hospital. Without productivity improvement, the cost of health care will become prohibitive and, in turn, quality health care in sufficient quantity could become a luxury affordable to only the affluent segments of society. With productivity improvement, the health care industry can do a more effective job of containing costs and providing a sufficient quantity and quality of health care for a larger portion of the population.

REFERENCES

1. Coile, R.C., Jr. *The New Hospital: Future Strategies for a Changing Industry.* Rockville, Md.: Aspen Publishers, 1986, p. 5.

2. Gray, S.P., and Steffy, W. *Hospital Cost Containment Through Productivity Management.* New York: Van Nostrand Reinhold, 1983, p. 1.

3. Beer, M., et al. *Human Resource Management: A General Manager's Perspective.* New York: Free Press, 1985.

4. Ibid.

5. Hackman, J.R., and Oldham, G.R. *Work Redesign.* Reading, Mass.: Addison-Wesley, 1980.

6. Dyer, W.G. *Team Building: Issues and Alternatives.* Reading, Mass.: Addison-Wesley, 1977.

7. Brisley, C.L. "Work Sampling." *Industrial Engineering Handbook,* edited by H.B. Maynard. 2d ed. New York: McGraw-Hill, 1963.

8. Lawler, E.E. III. *Pay and Organization Development.* Reading, Mass.: Addison-Wesley, 1981.

9. Winer, B.J. *Statistical Principles in Experimental Design.* 2d ed. New York: McGraw-Hill, 1981.

Index

Notes

Notes

Notes

Notes

Notes

Notes

Notes

Notes

Notes

Notes

Notes

Notes

Notes

Notes

Notes

Notes